Wardlife

The Apprenticeship of a Young Writer
as a Hospital Clerk

Andrew Steinmetz

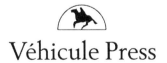

Véhicule Press

Acknowledgements

Thanks to Nicolas and Birgitta Steinmetz, for never panicking.

Thanks also to: Alen Matic, Michael Harris, Fred Biggar, Steve Sinclair, Louis Dussault, and Clara Gabriel; Good Cookies, Rosanne Cash, Big Star; John and Nancy Tarasuk; the pear and milk drink at Open Da Night, and to whatever was on tap at Bar Bobard in the winter of '95.

Special thanks to Simon Garamond for taking this off my hands.

Véhicule Press acknowledges the on-going support of The Canada Council for the Arts.

Cover design: J.W. Stewart
Cover photograph: Thomas Leon Königsthal, Jr.
Cover imaging: André Jacob
Interior design and imaging: Simon Garamond
Printing: AGMV-Marquis Inc.

CANADIAN CATALOGUING IN PUBLICATION DATA

Steinmetz, Andrew
  Wardlife

ISBN 1-55065-121-8

  1. Hospital patients. 2. Hospital wards. I. Title.
II. Title: Wardlife.

RA965.6.S84 1999   362.1'1   C99-900788-2

Published by Véhicule Press, Montréal, Québec
www.vehiculepress.com

Distributed by General Distribution Services.
Printed in Canada on alkaline paper.

For Marianne
and for Jill

Leech *n.* (arch., poet., or joc.) physician, healer; *leech craft*, art of healing. **Leech** *n.* aquatic blood-sucking worm of class Hirudinea, esp. *Hirudo medicinalis* formerly much used medicinally for bleeding.

The Concise Oxford Dictionary, 7th ed.

That was how it was. And I nodded to the family. They knew nothing about it, and, had they known, would not have believed it. To write prescriptions is easy, but to come to an understanding with people is hard.

Franz Kafka, from *A Country Doctor*
(Translated by Willa and Edwin Muir)

Contents

ICU

Report. T died last night. Ischemic bowel: dead tissue down below, zero bloodflow, no oxygen, rotting, gangrene. That's the story.

I am the unit co-ordinator. The UC. Non-medical staff. A civilian among the troops. I sit with a dummy terminal beside a telephone with more keys than an accordion. I'm the one who relays messages, calls for reinforcements. A kind of in-house, on-the-scene dispatcher. A blood-test and X-ray requisition distributing machine. Someone who sits on the guard rail between sickness and health, whistles while he works, someone who knows as little magic as medicine and practices the authority of neither.

Our location is the nth floor of the X pavilion. The unit has two sides, north and south wings, seven private and three shared rooms, space for twenty-one. It's newly built. Paint, floor tiles, monitors, and beds. A state of the art module. Everything is detachable, on wheels, electric, or battery operated. A nursing station with raised pink counter tops, sparse, generic as a fast food chain restaurant. The nurses, residents, students, and staff doctors thrive on the spaciousness and over-all newness of the place; it seems to have a placebo effect on everyone. Other wings in this hospital are drab and dilapidated, by comparison a gulag where time has not visited since the Quiet Revolution. Sometimes I am asked to go work on one of those floors, and I won't go. I stay here in the ICU, a place of witness where every heart rhythm and urine output is monitored, measured, and charted.

A controlled environment, a safe place where I fill a permanent part-time slot on a third-echelon pay scale.

Dr. G and Dr. B stand before me behind the raised counter, only heads showing, chins planted, making chit-chat like two swimmers resting at poolside. One of them is coming on call, the other going off. Together they review cases, shoot the breeze. In Room 34, bed 2 is an 80-year-old lady ... in Room 34, bed 3 is a 40-year-old gentleman ... in Room 50, bed 4 is a young fellow who came in with pneumonia. Between brief histories, the talk is about the next rotation, concern about the vacation schedule, research projects, and a local human rights case.

Come inside Room 50. A tag-team of nurses and orderlies are working steadily on Bed 3, emptying buckets of water into an open IV bag hung high on a pole, a reservoir. What are they doing? They call it a gastric lavage. Pronounced *lah-vah-ge*. A tummy bath. It's a complicated set-up, an aqueduct arrangement of conduits and channels, plastic tubing, parallel lines connected to a double-barrel syringe.

F is the man in bed number 3. He is what all the fuss is about. Tubing inserts by way of the mouth, deep, deep down into the stomach of F.

How does it work? Explanation: each pump of the double syringe, water is forced into F's intestines and simultaneously, bloody fluids are evacuated from the right-side cartridge into a metal, champagne-style bucket below bed level. And when the syringe is drawn, bloody-water rises up the line from F's stomach and fresh water is drawn from the overhanging IV bag into the left-side cartridge.

It's a question of equal and opposite reactions, pressure equilibrium, life and death.

F is conscious while the allied health team attend to this washing up. Fluids are flowing in and out, ebb and flow, rising and falling. Even while blood is being suctioned from his stomach, our man is receiving multiple transfusions. Good money after bad? It depends on who you play cards with.

Held on his side, F grunts, then vomits. Plugs are glued to his chest and his heart rate appears as a creeping electric wave on a terminal screen above the headboard. A hypnotic signal, like lightning thrown sidelong through water.

What's next? The gastro-enterology consult.

A scope is done and from their end it doesn't look good. The in-house GI resident rings home and instructs the cook to hold supper—"yes, again!"— she's stuck in the ICU with a major bleed.

So am I, stuck. Monday to Friday, 18:30 to 21:30. It's a jungle in here.

Time for my evening rounds of delivering labels and stationery to the nurses. They call me the professor, the way my arm cradles the load like a stack of term papers. I walk my beat, room to room, pausing to talk with staff and visitors. It's late now, my shift is almost over, so this is a social routine.

I meet Y, graphic designer, cyclist, nurse. He asks me how to spell firm, as in "a firm bowel movement." He's doing his charting.

"F-i-r-m," I tell him.

"So what about f-e-r-m," he counters.

"No such thing. There is an f-e-r-n, but that's the plant".

"But what about a company firm?"

"No," I say, "a corporate firm and a firm bowel movement are the same f-i-r-m."

This is too much for Y. He shakes his head. It's typical. He rolls his eyes, smirks, here it comes—see there, a quiet joy breaking his mask, for he has just diagnosed in me a disadvantage he is glad to be living without—the clumsy tool that is English.

We are friends, we connect on a lot of things, music, films, authors, but by this example all that Y has forever held as true about the local linguistic lines has been confirmed, that is, the way I think and he thinks are different — irreconcilable as, say, my English and his French. And as for me, suddenly the whole language debate in Quebec, as well the zero deficit target commandeered by our Premier, reduces to this: the grey area between a firm turd and the firm hand of business.

K is with us. He arrived on the unit several weeks ago. A symphony of symptoms, a case of general deterioration. K is the property of Vascular Surgery. Not much they can do for him. They gave him seven to ten days, but he's taken that and multiplied it many times over. Tonight I get news from down the line that K is *really* dying, all the experts agree, my informers from every level of the hospital strata, including the cleaning staff who feel these things as much as anyone.

K's wife stands at his bedside from morning to night. On guard, she is never seen sitting down. Her feet must swell. But I suppose she doesn't want to miss whatever it is that is going to happen when it happens. In the early evening, she is joined by two attractive young women: her daughters. They unfold around their mother, taking off jackets and laying them in a chair while they listen to their mother's synopsis of the day's events. He goes up and down hill, their father. It must be like following the yellow jersey rider in the Tour de France. And there also is a son, who lives out of town and who telephones frequently. Once a day the first week, twice a day now. When he calls, I put him through to his mother. I know him by voice. He knows mine.

K is thin as wire. He has one black foot, the tip of the iceberg.

"He won't be going anywhere," announces the Sheriff, our chief resident, who carries the responsibility of informing the staff assignment nurse about what we call here, the bed situation: who is well enough to go to the wards, who is unstable, who is beyond science, who is recovering nicely but must stay put.

Wardlife. P shuffles by the station, neck limp, head in full swing like incense at mass. Here he comes, threading a small congregation of lab-coated interns, he follows his course down the hall and back. His wife is a liver failure. She's in the OR. When she comes out she'll have graduated to the rank of a post-op liver. Here you are your procedure: she's a liver transplant, he's a heart transplant, he's a radical nephrectomy. Or, if you like, in shorthand, the familiar case: she's a liver, he's a heart.

P has oily grey hair, a square face, moist eyes, and is dressed in a V-neck sweater with no undershirt, tan trousers, black shoes. A smoker, 45–50 years; my guess. He wears that look of inadequacy to which men who live surrounded by a family of women commit themselves: doubtful, inadequate, a man who has worked a good while at a solitary trade, computers or engines, and now has been dropped—mid-stride —face to face with the uncertainties and vagaries of people.

P turns to me and asks for the time. I tell him. He shakes his shoulders and returns to his pre-occupation with measuring the length of the corridors. Again he returns and asks the time. I point to the clock behind me. Not much I can do about it. He understands. Our arms are tied. What can we do? We are not surgeons, these things take time.

To show him I am his ally, I put aside my work and pause, momentarily, gazing behind me at the clock. For an instant we are locked in the same world as together we stand and face the wall clock. Under our magnified stare, the second hand shivers under the glass, displaying slight hesitation before it passes over the next digit. Six. Seven. Eight. Nothing comes easy. Not the time, not the waiting. He goes away and double-checks with one of the nurses. Same thing. The nurse points to the clock and gestures, hand slicing the air, making some rough calculations.

P sits down, his feet start playing under the chair. Hand in lap, hunched but head held above his shoulders, he surveys us all, nurses, co-ordinator, doctors. Useless, next to useless. I watch him from behind the counter. An hour passes. I stamp some stationery. He wanders off, then he's back sitting. I check on him. His eyes migrate over my head to the clock pinned to the wall. Then they slide back down and gaze left towards the OR doors: sights set, a concentrated stare, invested with an act of will that could bend spoons.

She will come through those doors. Whatever real powers he possesses, he's got the right idea through those doors she will come, no other. They'll roll her in—his wife, the post-op liver—a team of personal trainers, the escort service, about forty years of post-secondary education between them. One to hold the IV bag aloft. One to push and one to guide the stretcher. One to monitor the heart monitor. And one of them will do her breathing, bag her while en route, until she's hooked up on machine air. The anaesthetist will check in later, and so will the surgeon, after washing up, to see his work.

I know the routine, P doesn't. I watch his stifled expression and keep watching until a look of fond nostalgia washes over his face. A shake of the head, a generous smile. What is it he is thinking? He must know something that I don't know.

Veronika, in her early sixties, Romanian, one of the night orderlies. Forty years of hospital service, only minor repairs. Growing old, grown old, wiping bums, folding sheets and bringing water. She wears a tight white blouse, a piece that billows below the waist, tennis style, circa Billy Jean King. Beside her co-workers, a parade of shiny males with greenhouse-grown biceps, Veronika is stringy meat, obsolete.

Veronika relies on me to relay overhead announcements. She's hard of hearing, something she could fix if she wasn't so stubborn, proud. Instead, she compensates the old way by asking a lot of questions.

"What did you hear just then? Room 46 calling?"

"It wasn't for you. They wanted Respiratory."

"So okay then, I'll go bring some bloods upstairs to the lab. If *they* call and think I'm not working, tell them I'm gone five minutes."

They, the nurses, don't like Veronika. The staff are always complaining about her, about her anaemic work ethic. The chorus goes: she's rude, she's stupid, she's lazy. There's some truth to this, but mostly it's spiteful chatter, automatic secretions. So many here are accused of labour sins. In a large institution like this, of multiple hierarchies and unions, with a frozen workforce set in permanent positions—like the citizens of Pompeii—it's unavoidable that character assassination should become a mode of settling accounts, a sport akin to game-hunting. Only in Veronika's case the team of prosecutors are especially belligerent. Christ, can they be mean. It seems to be another instance of cruelty in the world, a micro-crisis with a history of grand social complexity.

It feels wrong to pity her, like a trap, but I do. What's wrong with me? I don't usually get involved in these things, office politics, compassion famines. So why now? Why defend V, why plead her case? Is this the only way to keep myself from slipping in amongst the mob?

Outside each private room sits a nurse on a stool before a raised table making notes, they call them Progress Notes. Illness narratives, patient as pilgrim. They measure and chart, administer and observe. I need a spot like that to get some good work done. Five hundred words a day. A high table. Discreet, quiet, no disturbances. And perfect lighting, no shadows.

The ICU is a bright oasis of calm compared to other units. Passing through the hall, passing doorways and looking in, the signs of life are few, among the machinery and tubing, the Cadillac-sized electric beds, inflatable heating blankets, blood pressure cuffs, lights and Christmas decorations, prongs and switches. It's difficult to discern the human from the machine, detect where one ends and the other begins. On a night like this, walking the halls, humming some Mozart, it's easy enough to pretend that everyone is tucked in and sleeping, having sweet dreams as they should be: they are not ill, no, only tired, as ones their age ought to be at eight-thirty at night.

What breaks this aura of peace and tranquillity is the suctioning of someone in Room 50, the tight sucking of saliva and phlegm and sputum, like you get at the dentist, except here they vacuum right down into the lungs, left lung, right lung.

Just how a wolf howling may destroy the impression of a sleeping forest in the winter. How you suddenly feel cold and notice darkness falling.

Report, change of shift: Mr. ___'s son was here …
tried to be strong but he broke down after a family
meeting. He said it was hard to see his father that
way… leave him as a 'No Ninety-nine' … hasn't been
walking since December. Mrs. ___ is allowed to eat
today, fluids, zero vomiting in the last 24 hours … no
family over the weekend and she's upset. Mrs. ___ …
fine … a bed bath yesterday. Mr. ___ one of the
residents came through early … D/C IV, start on fluids
today … on a sliding scale … no colostomy … doing
extremely well post-operatively … pain management
fine … a CT in the a.m. … nothing else left … frustrated
because she can't talk. That's about it, every one else
is coasting, have a good weekend. By the way, did
you hear? Cirque de Soleil is in town, at the Old
Port … we're going to bring the children.

They are wrapping a body in 34. The body bag, made from a tough, semi-transparent plastic, is like the ones used to protect dress suits during travel. And I guess this body is starting out on a journey. Watching the nurse and orderly do up the man in Room 34, my mind summons up images of all the other wrappings I've witnessed today. Like the contents of my felafel sandwich, wrapped in pita, then wrapped in wax paper. How the server held the sandwich in his fist, and cinched the paper wrapping, before handing it over the counter-top. Like the flowers outside the Pine avenue florist wrapped in cellophane cones. The silence, wrapped around the family of the expired man inside Room 34.

I call the transport team to come collect. They wheel in a blue plastic carriage covered over with a bed sheet. It looks like they built the thing in the garage out of what was lying around, but it's the real thing. Standard issue. My great-aunt who survived post-war Berlin told me once how the people made wagons by tying together pieces of broken furniture and bicycle wheels with wire and cloth, to carry wood for heating from the Tiergarten. She described how even the old looked foolish, childlike, pushing those makeshift wagons along grand avenues lined with sawed-off tree stumps.

The transport team on morgue duty always travels in twos. When they arrive on the unit, first off they must sign the death book. Every ward has one. Usually a black binder, pasted with a fat sticker that reads DEATH BOOK. Our thrift-store binder lacks the dignity of a heavy, fat ledger.

"Where do I sign? Here? Just my initials? Or the whole thing? Ask that guy? Let's ask him."

That guy is me. They are the transport team. And these are their questions.

These questions are not easy to answer because they are always the same, and because I have answered them many, many times, and because the protocol never changes. But everybody seems to dumb down around a dead body. No one wants to go wrong with the dead.

These days, when there's a pick-up, I lay the death book open on the counter, as I have done tonight, and hide out in the clean utility room when I hear the transport team bang through the swing doors at the end of the corridor. I leave them alone and let them sign where they want and how they want. Full name or initials, date, time. And then, after they leave, I come back out and check if they have taken away the right body. The death book I do not verify. I slap it shut and put it back in the drawer. Done.

Now here comes a delivery from a Chinese restaurant and he wants to know who ordered General Tao. Not me, one of the residents, I guess. I plug an announcement on the overhead. It won't be long, I tell the man. He nods and takes a step back from the counter, looks left, then right, checking the place out. Not his regular drop off, but no sweat, all he must to do is collect the $12.50 and hop back into his car. He can do that, he can wait. It's warm in here. And anyway, the nurse over there, who keeps coming by to ask why Cardiology haven't responded to her page, she's not bad looking.

Reminds me of the year I worked as a busboy at Chows, a Chinese restaurant on Dorval avenue. That was in 1981. Because I worked Friday nights, I missed my share of school dances. That was bad. But at the end of my shift I got a free meal and all evening I was allowed egg rolls and won ton soup. A big deal when you're 16 and suburban. And I remember Mrs. Lee, aged 70 or so, who used to grind meat and prepare the rolls in the basement. A cellar, not a basement. It was frigid and dark and she wore leather gloves. I wonder why I never questioned what a woman the age of my grandmother was doing at midnight in a cellar on Dorval avenue. It seemed so normal and it was. I suppose I already knew about first, second, and third worlds, and the class strata, and assumed it was her lot, a fair compromise for being Chinese, an immigrant. Could I have accepted that already? Sure, I could have. I did.

Mr. Lee, her husband, washed dishes with me. Mr. Lee and I communicated by a series of primitive hand gestures, hand-puppet theatre. We kept it simple. Of course there was no sensitive information to relay, we were not a multidisciplinary team back then. He dried and I washed, he washed and I dried. That's all we needed to get straight.

The clock display window on my phone reads 19:34, 19:35. I drifted. To my right two residents are chatting.

"Did you order?" I ask them.

"Nope, must have been Medicine," they respond. "What is it anyway?" they ask the delivery person.

"General Tao," I put in.

"We'll take it," they offer.

"Twelve-fifty," says the driver, who steps up and places the stapled, oil stained paper bag on the nursing station counter.

Now everybody is happy. The residents have their chicken and I've got a clean plate, nobody left waiting in the hallway.

"How is it?" I ask. I feel somewhat responsible.

"It's gross," says one. "But a good kind of gross."

All is quiet in the ICU. Still Life. Hewlett Packard printer humming at my elbow, a cooling fan stirring inside the metal cavity. Spacelabs cardiac output recorder is whining and beeping. It needs more paper. Forget it. It's impossible to feed the rolls into those things. Telephone napping at 18:30. Clock display window: the colon between 18 and 30 is blinking, on, off, on, off, on, off. Is it trying to warn me about something?

Last night we had a 52-year-old gentleman join us. Something of a celebrity around here. He hunted himself, a rifle, close range: hooked his toe on the trigger and tucked the barrel under his chin like a napkin. A foolproof strategy. Any dummy could do it, not this one though. He fired off target and blew away his jaw bone, leaving him without a tongue to explain the history of his disease to the psychiatry resident.

S. Room 50, bed 5. All aboard, all aboard.

My brother Oren passes behind the raised counter and I watch him come out the other end, thin, tall, tired, stooped. He's a vascular surgeon. Ten, eleven, I don't know how many years to become one, if you count undergraduate prerequisite courses, medical school, a residency in general surgery, then a vascular fellowship. I was in high school when he disappeared into the machinery, university, a marriage, then children. We've grown apart, but only like fingers off the one single hand. There are whole summers between us going back to the days before either of us mastered our multiplication tables. August in the Eastern Townships, our fields, the forests, sun, pond water. We played soccer using stumps as goal posts. Fishing, building forts, damming streams. He's done that and I've done that. If he was running, tripped, and fell, there was a good chance that I would be following, then have tripped and fallen right there on the ground beside him. All those years together, and so much of what happened to one of us, happened to us all, brothers and sister. We lived practically the same lives. Identical experiences. And now he is someone I love without ever telling him so. He visits the unit to settle accounts with medical students, and to visit his post-ops. He is well liked, respected, by staff and patients, for being fair and thorough. I'm actually proud of him in a way I never thought possible. It was he who got me this job in the first place. At least twice a week we cross paths, big brother, little brother, surgeon, clerk, we both have our roles whenever we meet. Here in the ICU our conversations cut a swath through concentric circles, outwards from hospital trivia to family stuff, stories about our children. Nothing new is learned during these brief exchanges. There is no need. Ours is a broad language.

"How are things?"

"Not bad. How's the writing?"

"Coming along."

It's our twice a week check-up, that's all. Routine follow-up procedure.

Tomorrow is another day and today is tomorrow. P has a friend, D, whose wife is in with cancer of something. We say CA—as in Chartered Accountant. Mrs. D is a picture. Bald. Bruised. Welts. She is one for whom an X-ray would do more justice. Her eyes, narrow, dry, defeated, betray a mixture of disappointment and shame. Not social shame, but animal, innate.

She has a look that is familiar around here. The features of one who will die a slow hospital death. An insidious process. A process that echoes Robert Frost's description of a wood pile and what he called the slow, smokeless fire of decay.

P and D are a pair: married to women near death. Their wedding vows have come back to haunt them, in sickness and in health ... the ritual is real, their words, made flesh. This place has become an old haunt for them by week's end. And after passing each other in the hall these last days, pacing, now and then imposing an apologetic greeting—an embarrassed gesture, as if to say: sir, I know that if my wife were not as sick, yours also would not be so badly off —as of this night the two have broken with decorum and started up a conversation. The hell with it all, if just for *this* minute. They have given up on fair-play, on trying to make any sense of it, and turned: a friendship awoken with a single touch on the shoulder.

They are calling for me in Room 42. L and T, two nurses. They need my help. It can't be serious.

Room 42 means Q. An epileptic. An OD, smorgasbord: what was under the sink, in the mirror cabinet, and behind the bar. She's slipping into brain-dead-dom.

"Can you help us?"

Q has a tube down her nose.

L and R are preparing the solution, a dose, measuring a cup of water, squeezing a tube of black ooze. Liquid charcoal. It's messy stuff, arts and crafts. On the bed table lies a Toomey, the shotgun of the syringe family. Toomeys are used to stuff charcoal down the NG, the naso-gastric tube, and into the belly to neutralize toxic juices.

L and R are not sure how much water to add, how much charcoal. Two to one, or three to one? What's the ratio? That's why they called me in, to read them the instructions—in English, only—off the side of the bottle.

"How did this get into Quebec?" L asks. She's flustered. "It should be in French to sell it in Quebec. That's the law."

No one denies this, I don't. The law is the law and this time it makes good sense. She's not angry at me but at someone who I feel is standing over my shoulder, flying a flag over the Plains of Abraham.

I hold up the bottle, just like a soup can or a cereal box, and read, happy to be of help.

Update: K maintains a course of steady deterioration, but we can still see him. He's not invisible. Daughters and wife serenade. Ukrainian hymns. Beautiful harmonies leak down the hallway. Voices laced with feeling, laced together. They strike a chord in me. I switch off the radio, a news documentary about the snipers of Sarajevo. I cup my hands over my ears to capture their singing voices, isolated from the hi-tech breathing of our small chorus of life machines.

The snipers of Sarajevo, the guns of Beirut. Memory is a broad continuum. What was it? The late seventies?

In the back of our station wagon crossing the Champlain Bridge, a radio playing—in those days it was always Cross Country Checkup—that's when the sound of real sniper fire first got through to me. I was lying on my back, knees up, marooned in the anonymity of a Plymouth, crouched low behind the back seats and aware of a dark, nuclear density of shopping bags, parcels, and suitcases.

"Beirut," I heard them say two seats up. "Imagine if we lived in Beirut ..."

My parents always wanted us, the children, to imagine we lived some place else, in another country, but I couldn't imagine those things then, and I didn't know the city of Beirut from the suburb of Baie d'Urfé. My universe was the present moment: a black sky, a few stars, flickering lights. Shadows floated across the car ceiling like an enemy moving along the walls. I lay there, head on a pillow, wondering, staring out the side windows at the night sky and sniper fire ricocheted off bombed-out buildings in the left-side speakers.

"Are you okay back there?"

What could happen to me back there? My mother was a constant worrier. My sister, now, asleep. My father driving, my brothers playing Who Am I? Fielding questions, yes and no answers. And the back of their heads were like the back of heads of people at movies. Everyone faced forward, out the front windshield our car lights sprayed into the darkness.

I felt myself begin to drift, slipping in and out, off to sleep. Someone turned the radio dial. Static, dead space, programing. Choral music. Handel. A Coronation Anthem. My heart started bleeding, then.

A man from a courier company in a tight-fitting, brown vest enters the ICU pushing a trolley loaded with boxes labelled Fragile and This Side Up.

"The leeches," announces he, and asks me to sign.

I have the authority, I suppose, to sign for segmented worms.

"Here," he points to a spot, "and here."

"There you go."

He takes possession of the sales slip and glances at my ID badge and nods his head, slowly. I can see he's not satisfied with our exchange. Something is amiss. It doesn't seem right to him, what do you need leeches for in a hospital? That's a question I'm asking myself, but first I gotta get rid of this secret agent.

"Is that it?" I inquire, adding starch: "Thank you." You can leave. I sound firm. Soon as he's gone, I turn to the assistant head nurse.

"What are these for?"

"Room 50, bed 5."

Beside her elbow is a junk pile of erasers, pencils, coloured pens, liquid ink. Deeply bored, she's working on the staff schedule.

"They use them in Plastics. Don't worry, the doctor will know."

I go find a hand trolley, load up the boxes, and wheel them into Room 50. I'll get to the bottom of this.

"The leeches," I announce, taking the courier's strategy of nonchalance for a good one.

"Put them over by the table," instructs nurse T. He's busy with Bed 4. Bed 4 is being suctioned.

I wait in the corner of the room, finger-drumming the cardboard.

"They're for Vascular." T shouts from across the room.

"Don't they use them in Plastics, too?" I feign a casual familiarity with the *Hirudo medicinalis*, that's their Christian name for those in the know.

"Plastics, Vascular, whatever—they suck blood."

Fair enough. He's not an expert.

After doing some background reading on aquatic blood-sucking worms, I discovered something interesting about the therapeutic value of leeches. It appears their saliva is not just any idiot's drool, but contains a wonder substance that anaesthetises the wound area (sharp teeth make a Y shaped incision), dilates blood vessels, and prevents blood from clotting. Three-in-one, nature's formula.

What does this have to do with Bed 5? Bed 5 had surgery, something was removed, something was added. Plastics engineered the reconstruction process, now it's Vascular's turn to get the blood circulating through the tissue flap. Enter the lowly leeches. Their dominant behaviour is to suck. Sucking relieves venous congestion in replanted tissue.

I hang around and help T set up the aquarium. I'm happy to do it. I never had fish at home so this is something new. Opening up the box, I wonder if the aquarium comes with sand, coral, a miniature sea castle. Or if that stuff's extra.

T and I get busy. We open the big box first, labelled Fragile, and pull out a glass rectangle. I get some water. I fill up one of those champagne buckets they use to collect chest drainage fluids.

"Are you sure they like this water?" What I mean is, should we use saline, instead?

"No. This is good." T is solid on the living conditions of the *Hirudo medicinalis*.

Next we open This Side Up. It contains the leeches. I don't know how they know the difference, up, down, underwater.

The leeches are packaged in a tough plastic container. They don't look active. But remember, sucking is their dominant behaviour, not swimming.

While we play, Bed 5 is sleeping. At least I think she's sleeping. I've never really understood the difference between sleeping and being unconscious, or in a coma.

We're quiet, we hurry to get everything set before she wakes up. That way it will be a surprise.

At the bottom of the box, I retrieve a bag of white powder. Nutrients? The bag isn't labelled.

"It must have to do with the pH, maybe it's salt or something."

Either one of us could have said that. We mix it in. They're only leeches.

From Spain: Gina, the 59-year-old service assistant. Dressed in terminal black, in mourning—she's the one who anointed me *Andrei The Lazy*.

Gina is on the ward tonight because her husband, a skinny, elegant man of 60-plus, is in for a heart operation. She keeps herself busy by cutting paper labels into squares. We use them to identify blood tubes. Vacutainers. She's not on duty, she could read a magazine instead, but a hospital employee over 30 years, she's one of those old-school workers who feel loyalty to this place, even in their time off. Even in the era of budget cuts, staff reductions, and cute new mission statements.

"You could knit me a sweater instead ..."

End of shift, I'm leaving. Her husband is still in the OR. They're doing a job on him. I say goodnight, she frowns.

"Andrei, my mother only trained me to build socks. Don't be so stupid ... you are really something lazy."

Gina is the matriarch of the blue collar workers and clerks, the cleaners of this palace, the *lumpen* proletariat. These square feet are her domain. Standing under five feet tall, proud as a barrel, she likes to admonish me, my youth, my New Worldness. In return, I enjoy the attention of her displaced affection, the certainties of an old world ruler. She was born on an island in a village without a doctor, she makes her own wine and can build socks, and because I don't seem to know how to do any one of these things and all I do is stamp papers and stab at the keyboard—because, because—she concluded long ago that I'm wasting somebody's time and somebody's money.

"You do what?—All the time, Andrei?"

That's a good way to put it. I do do what. A unit co-ordinator—what I do—she will never see *that*, never have one of those back on her island.

Report. Mrs. E passed away. She expired. DD-MM-YY. "Don't you remember, the nice lady in Room 32? Come on, the one with mets. Remember her?"

Sorry but I don't—around here metastatic cancer doesn't narrow the field. I follow the progress and deterioration of a number of patients, but not all.

As with the healthy, so with the ill, some people strike me, some don't, and it never makes much sense why I do or I don't, why I am generous towards some, indifferent to others. But we all have our limits, vows, and houses to keep in order, and you can only look after so much, lend a hand only so often. Should I pin it down to that? Dismiss it? As when the day is done, chances are the books are balanced, you feel fine, maybe a little irritated with something or someone—you forget which—but overall you feel a certain acceptance of yourself without ever needing to read the small print or enter into the arithmetic. Does that sound good? Good enough.

Just went to deliver a blood gas result in Room 48 and found Dr. R, a friend of mine—we shared some arak last summer on a balcony—inserting a black tube into D's anus. A sigmoidoscopy. That's what he's up to. The black tube, similar to a garden hose, blows air and inflates the colon as it progresses up the canal, while a camera implant takes snapshots of the intestinal walls. He must be on the look-out for a bleed, an ulcer or a polyp, something of that nature.

I had one done myself, so I know how it feels to be hyper-inflated. You can actually detect the progress of the tubing as it winds in, up through the alimentary canal by way of Upper Egypt. A funny feeling. Invasive, they say. This is medicine *sans frontières*. From his end, the doctor manipulates and twists the hose, guided by the video display. Of course, these days no one sets foot anywhere on the planet without video. In my case, since I was good and compliant, they allowed me to watch the live telecast. I lay on my tummy, head turned sharp left to catch the action on a twenty-inch Sony.

And good heavens, what a view. Here's proof: beauty *is* only skin deep. Otherwise, the inside may be more interesting than the outside, after all. The scenery was unearthly. I half expected stalactites. Who knows, down there, they might discover hieroglyphics that pre-date our earliest fossil records.

What I saw was not unlike a movie clip wherein the police lower themselves down man-holes into the sewage system, holding awkward lamps, and chase criminals through a labyrinth of semi-flooded passageways.

Didn't enjoy that. One helluva fart when it's done.

In come a surgery team on rounds. The chief resident leads the way, followed closely by his brood, a mix of junior residents and students hugging clipboards and nibbling Styrofoam cups. Patient rounds, these are imprinting grounds. A ragged bunch, their circadian rhythms hang on them like loose underwear. No surprise, the hours they keep are ridiculous. I wonder how their endogenous clocks are set?

Circling the unit, going room to room, they meet up with another lost patrol. Green surgery, meet blue surgery. They go by different colours like street gangs, but they're all alike.

The two chiefs shake hands, receive each other and review notes. They exchange academic journal citations and begin telling staff stories, which are cautionary tales about their own bosses—staff surgeons with end-stage personality disorders. Staff stories are crowd pleasers, good for a laugh, formulated OR sitcoms linked by to-be-continued freeze-frames.

Meanwhile, a call comes in at the desk. A page for General Surgery. There's a case in the Emergency. A possible appendix. Somebody better check it out. Who's on call? Green or blue? It's six o'clock. Negotiations ensue. They decide to dispatch a green student down to the ER on reconnaissance. In return, the student appears wounded. It's a bum mission. Scut work, they call it. She was hoping to split for home after rounds.

After the student leaves, things loosen up. Green and blue stand a face, at ease, chatting.

"Did you see Hole last weekend?"

"No man, I couldn't go."

I know most of these doctors, fellows, residents, interns, students, their politics, religion, sexuality, all obvious things. They pass years in the hospital, learning, training, serving. It's a gradual metamorphosis. A brainwash. Sleep deprived and overworked, they earn their stripes like members of some fanatical cult. And by the time one of them becomes chief of something there's a good chance I will have squared off in a squash court with them, if they play squash, that is.

Looking over the group—the assembled humanity of green and blue surgery—I notice what I notice: hijab, kippot, Doc Martens, a péquiste, federalists, and a grab bag of secular materialists. The team of '99. They're happy, they get along, no one's fighting. They have hope, a good thing going—just so as long as everybody gets their own operating room time, and no one from outside occupies their ICU beds. Then nobody's going to get hurt. And nobody's going to try to hurt anybody.

I saw Gina in the waiting room on my way in. Her husband is recovering from his operation, sleeping in Room 34. Knock on wood.

I'm working on the CVT side today. Cardiovascular and Thoracic Surgery. Heart transplants, lobectomies, bypasses. That's the stuff.

"How many cabbages?" You hear that often, our measure of productivity. "How many for tomorrow?"

A cabbage, or CABG, is a coronary artery bypass graft. It sounds like something a civil engineer is trained to build—a roadway, an overpass—to improve circulation on the main motorways.

"No cabbages on Tuesdays," I disappoint. Market talk. Supply and demand. They'll have to settle for a Triple A. An abdominal aortic aneurysm. They're major league. My brother does those.

When a cabbage returns from surgery, that is a sight to behold. Rolled by the nursing station, they are so peaceful under anaesthetic, cocooned and wrapped in blankets and pain killers, their eyes glisten. The lids are closed with a gel for protection against the bright OR lights. It appears that they've been slimed: in an altered state, undergoing a stage of metamorphosis. Eyes in their sockets, larvae in the grub state. The first time you see one it's disturbing, until now, now I can walk into Room 86 like a professional, where there might be five cabbages in a row, and I can move bed to bed, hand out stationery, deliver test results, even talk with the families, without anything showing on the outside that I feel on the inside.

49

I walk into Room 50 and look: a limp penis and catheter, a mouth taped to hold an air tube. S, our attempted suicide on his back, spread like a fried egg.

I've been off for the long weekend. Three days in the country. My head's somewhere else, I gotta get back into the swing of things.

Supine, covers off, S's belly protrudes, a hairy, grassy knoll. Like one of those rounded hills you come across in England's Lake District. In the region of Windermere, where, in late eighteenth and early nineteenth centuries, the peripatetic poet Wordsworth set out in the mornings to power-walk and chat with leech gatherers. What a long way that is from here, "Lines Composed a Few Miles above Tintern Abbey." I studied that poem under Professor Swain at McGill and I remember especially—*The still, sad music of humanity*—six words, impressed on my imagination.

The nurses try to keep things decent, but repeatedly the covers slide off, down the slope and onto his knees, so that S's metropolitan area is on display.

Professor Arnold Swain. He was chairman, or vice-chairman of the English department. A man travelling beyond his late fifties with the visionary company of Keats, Wordsworth, and Shelley. Milton was another of his favourites. At McGill, Professor Swain taught a four-hundred level, three-credit seminar. Twice a week I joined his class, a handful of students, we assembled our intellects around a wood table in the seminar room, a room with sore lighting, and Professor Swain read aloud to us, his apostles, descriptions of Adam and Eve from *Paradise Lost*.

A liberal arts education can be a terrible thing to remember.

Professor Swain practised an oblique sense of humour that was lost on many, self-important and serious as we were—spellbound initiates—especially one boy from Toronto who I remember was unusually agitated as he was undergoing the natural selection process of becoming a Rhodes Scholar. Anyhow, I remember that once Professor Swain related to us, how, long into his marriage, after several children and station wagons, he discovered himself in a kitchen reading *Paradise Lost* aloud to his wife—softly, from behind, into her ear—while she washed dishes. In reality not much of a joke but an odd image, and one that has stuck with me over the years.

He's been intubated. They tubed him. They set the pipe down his airway and taped it.

I feel nostalgic tonight as I do my rounds, on a summer night: even though this place is sealed shut, ventilated, and scrubbed clean with monster detergents, you can feel summer inside. There's a special quality of light. A glow. A lightness in the air as I go on my way, room to room, dreaming about *Paradise Lost* and remembering Professor Swain. I haven't read any poetry in months, but back then—back ten years — I was under the influence of Professor Swain, of his precious Keats and Shelley, poets who kept me writing term papers throughout my undergraduate years and right into graduate school at University of Toronto, where, under the guidance of a tutor who has since died of AIDS, I wrote my final paper, What Does a Poet Do? I guess I had the same questions about poets as Gina has about unit co-ordinators.

After graduate school, I moved back to Montreal. I had no plans. I wasn't doctorate material. I played in a few bands and I started writing my own stories. A writer's apprenticeship is an intensely private thing. Lonely, full of doubts, and, in this age, undeniably pretentious. But already, I knew, I was on the trail of something. I went to Europe and travelled for months and did nothing but stare out the window of the train. Travel, they say, is an excuse for being. If that's so, well then I have been.

A penis and catheter, a mouth taped to hold a breathing tube.

When my rail pass expired at the end of the summer, I returned home and over the next years, a dynamic evolved. Only when I was reading did I feel that I was progressing, improving myself, getting somewhere, but getting where? In Professor Swain's class I studied poems like they were maps. The more difficult the writing, the greater the hidden treasure of meaning. I kept reading and following, so it felt, on a path of imminent revelation. I finally came across an essay by Borges and in it, that phrase, about the imminence of a revelation, about the aesthetic experience being essentially a tease, a fever, a phenomenon that can run you ragged as it did Shelley's Alastor. The same phenomenon that kept me staring out the window of a train from Budapest to Lisbon.

I look back over the years now and see shadows falling differently. I see Professor Swain on tenure track, a moveable sidewalk—scholar squeezed beside scholar, worn, tired Magi—with a long face, drooping earlobes, cheeks patched rose, and eyes searching everywhere with a gaze tinged with sadness. What is it in his eyes, what grave concern? A metaphysical appeal, imminence of a revelation?

Still, the sad music. A penis, a catheter, a breathing tube. This is not the wonderful world of Disney.

Room 48. G is septic which sounds pretty awful. A condition related to the putrefactive destruction of tissues, that is, their decomposition. By whom? By what? By disease-causing bacteria and their toxins. Septicaemia is blood poisoning.

G is stewing, stewing in his own bad blood.

There's a photograph of him, from better days, on the bed table. The families do that to remind the staff that their loved ones are loved ones.

G's son is in for a visit. Baseball cap, baggy pants. They explain to him what sepsis is, that's how I learn too.

I overheard the boy telling the resident that his father was a fighter, "he's a tough one ... oh no, never, never gives up that one ... not him, tough as nails."

Then I saw the resident nod, sure. Whatever you say, kid. He was diplomatic about it, he listened. He cocked his head, and in a mechanical gesture had one ear follow the boy's voice while his eyes kept roving elsewhere, soliciting other signals.

It was sad to see it all, to know it all from seeing it all before.

No matter what the boy says, he can't convince anybody around here that his father is going to live into the next month, when residents and staff doctor change over at the beginning of another teaching rotation.

A break in the action. I warm up a cup of tea for U, an old face I remember from my days on 9 Surgery. I rarely have the time to perform civil acts. A slow shift like this is a welcome change, good for the soul.

U is in with her husband. All I know about him is he has something called a jejunostomy tube, and it needs maintenance.

U is an elderly woman, let's say late sixties, early seventies. She has long braided hair, white-grey, like my own living grandmother has. Her eyes are sunken, but serene, and when she confers with the doctors, she treats the occasion with a manner of grace and a generosity and gentleness of spirit that more often characterizes moments between grandparents and their grandchildren.

I offer her a cup of tea and she smiles and clasps her hands around mine.

"Thank you for this," she says, still holding my hands.

"It's nothing," I say, although it feels like something. It does me good to do good, doctors must feel great.

"It's very kind."

She could build a civil society all by herself.

On my way in I passed by the waiting room and picked up a Coke. In one of the cubicles, a woman was kneeling on the floor. I had to step around her to get to a machine. She was wearing a hijab so I understood she wasn't looking for a lost earring. She was praying, facing the one ton, neon drink machine, a Western wonder.

You drop money, press a button, and a cold drink pops out, the real thing.

Later on I saw her again on the unit with a box of Smarties. It was written, I suppose. Those machines must have been a temptation, it's not for nothing that mosques don't bear icons. Standing in the hall, the Arab woman was in conference with a team of doctors. Her brother was the subject. And evidently there were communication problems, cultural barriers. Still, without a common language, god, or sitcom between them, they seemed to make out somehow.

At the desk, someone pointed: she's pushy and acts like a man, said one nurse, which she meant as a criticism I guess.

"It's cultural," said someone to our left.

"It's not cultural," replied the first nurse, annoyed, "women in their countries aren't allowed to do anything. So it's not cultural."

Then I guess it's personal.

The woman popped Smarties into her mouth while one doctor, a medical student with an uncanny resemblance to Mr. Bean, played out the scene of her brother with a breathing obstruction. Next, act two, scene two, the same doctor placed a pen between his lips and withdrew it, exhaling, and she shook her head in the negative. No, he didn't smoke or drink, read your Koran. That's good, he beamed, and placed a hand way up on her shoulder, while she stood there like the Tower of Babel itself. He held out his other arm and displayed his watch. Time. She understood that. Time will tell, inshallah.

I'm glad N is working tonight. He always shakes things up. A queen. A nurse. Bilingual, bisexual. My first shift in the ICU, he swung up behind me, gave me a bump, and whispered into my ear, "Watch out little fella, I'm the queen bee. One sting and you'll work for me!"

I was warned about him. Tonight we talk about movies and guardian angels. He wants to go work up north, in the Arctic, and make a pile of money but he can't, back home he's taking care of his father.

"No rest for the wicked," he sounds defeated.

His father has Alzheimer's, that is, Alzheimer's has his father.

"You mean the naked," I try to spin off something.

"What?"

"…no rest for the naked."

He likes that, laughs. Licks his lips. I guess I'm all right for a straight.

Veronika update. Situation: kindergarten. Veronika walks too slow, she takes long breaks, she comes in late, ignores the call bells, basically, she's a witch. Behind her back, they mock her accent, her gestures, all she is about. She is our own private Yugoslavia.

I've been watching Veronika, standing close, poised yet impotent, UN observer-like. I'm trying to find out what it is about her that inspires so much disdain, in some cases, outright repulsion. It's irrational. Mechanical, systematic. Under the microscope, what stands out is her blouse, a garment yellowed from wear. I keep coming back to that blouse again and again, Veronika and her blouse, Citizen Kane and Rosebud. It's worn, tight, thinned, her undergarments, themselves tired of the routine and weight, show through as they are—incompetent, no longer capable of the task for which they were designed. A metaphor for Veronika herself?

That's the kind of mind I have. Explain the obvious by the obscure, I'm always looking for material.

Funny that when you begin caring-despairing for someone like Veronika, and come close to opening up to their needs—needs and demands of a magnitude which engage your own reserves for compassion, and find them wanting—finally you reject the opportunity, as your system would reject a foreign organ. You find, instead, comfort in disparaging their wardrobe. And you find no great crime in that.

Waiting for a donor, for Godot, for the man. A month ago, we had a liver failure come stay with us. X was going toxic waiting for a donor. Finding a donor means getting hold of an intact corpse with the right blood type and shoe size match, and the wait can be long: waiting for Godot. To simplify matters, there is a professional group, a society of head-hunters with a wish list, who co-ordinate the delivery of refrigerated body parts (in red and white thermoses) by helicopter across the province and nation-wide. A good bet for a donor is a biker—they call them donor-cycles—or a young male: hence the man, in waiting for the man. Now if the donor is a local boy, our surgeons do their own harvesting and the head-hunters are left out of the loop. Harvesting is when the donor is spread out on the table like an evening laid out against the sky and surgeons, dressed like bandits in mask and gown, extract the gold and silver. The heart, lungs, kidney, liver. Anything that might go on ticking or pumping or filtering inside another body.

In the case of X, our liver, there was no match to be found and meanwhile our transplant candidate was failing, that is, dying. With no prospective donor on record, the patient signed a consent to have himself temporarily connected up to a pig's liver. It was to be a groundbreaking *porcedure*, an event, and the surgeons were going to perform it right here in the ICU, not in the OR. As I recall, there were two surgeons, and both were excited to carry out the procedure, giddy, like schoolboys, mischievous before exploding a frog. At one interval, I watched as they laid open a medical journal article on the nursing station counter, making diagrams and consulting over details, hesitating now before getting started, as if they were about to build a toy model from badly typed instructions, right there on the living room floor, on hands and knees, on Christmas morning.

The pig procedure, as we called it, was a great success. And the Pig Man, as became his in-house show name, benefited almost immediately from his partnership agreement. His blood was channelled through the porcine liver which performed like a swimming pool filter and reduced levels of toxicity in his blood. Ammonia levels. NH3 or NH2. I forget which. But I do remember our excitement, our nervous, greedy curiosity—mine and others', members of the staff—who watched from a side-window, secluded by a one-way mirror. It was none other than a medical science peep-show. And I remember, also, that someone made an off-colour joke about whether or not the pig man was Jewish and what that would mean.

Dr. C cradled the pig liver like a gerbil in his rubber-gloved palms. When the tubes were hooked up, pig liver to man, man to pig liver, the animal organ inflated with human blood.

That's fantastic, my conscience spoke. Simple mechanics. Elementary science. Everything is simple mechanics when you get right down to it, nothing odd about this … and this observation steadied things for me.

Within hours, X regained consciousness.

Everything worked fabulously. And the next day I received a phone call from a man who said he was the one who had slaughtered the pig in the lab, and he wanted to know how "the liver" was doing. I hesitated, and cupped my hand over the mouth piece, taken aback by the speaker's candid, though ambiguous, reference to the liver. Did he mean his liver—the pig liver? Or our liver—the transplant candidate?

I gave out no information, unsure if he was a crank. Or a reporter.

This just in. Room 42 has reached end-stage renal failure. Rarely do I get official word that anyone is dying. Our cases deteriorate with a phase four D or a stage three Y. They submit to complications, infested by a parasite of which no one understands the life-cycle, let alone how to spell the thing, it being of Latin etymology. The dying process is shrouded in mystery, in multifactorial mist, with more euphemisms than the Inuit have words for snow.

The doctors say S is difficult to wean, a definite no-no around here. It means he's not tolerating being taken off machine air. He's been pampered, I guess, by all the technology they showered him with. Spoilt rotten. To work things out, they've prescribed a private tutor, a respiratory therapist.

I love it here at night sometimes. A clean, well-lighted place. The brush of activity, precise tasks measure out the evening. I feel a certain dress of character, a positive hum, as though all my electrons were happily married. I feel as I felt when I was in Copenhagen one fine day: full, complete, free, an anthemic rising up of the self. And safety in numbers, I feel safe here where the team dressed in white lab-coats outnumber the skins, our few bedridden tonight. Everything will be taken care of, I feel sure there is enough time: to work, play, live; to take detours, dream, and eat dessert. There's time enough tonight to be the unit co-ordinator for three hours, to wipe clean my chair and the terminal screen, polish the telephone. These tireless objects, solid things with stable functions. Materials with half-lives you couldn't measure. This nursing station, well ordered, a luminous sanctuary. I imagine the two waiters and the drunk, deaf old man in Hemingway's story, as I go about wiping the counter-tops with a towel drenched in alcohol. That's the smell of clean. The antiseptic grave. It's not my job but doing it leaves a certain cleanness and order.

W died. Days ago, Dr. H and Dr. M opened her belly in Room 48. I looked in on my rounds and W's bowel was coiled up on her stomach like a cat. A clock, opened and the mechanical innards had popped out. Blood sausage. How long can you keep that out before it spoils? I sneaked a second glance on a return visit. There was something diabolical about it, obscene, I had to see more—not to look, but to verify what I had seen.

On closing W, the doctors sewed a white zipper with plastic teeth and synthetic borders into her abdomen. Better than stitches, the zipper was thought up to facilitate repeat access to her bowels. Earlier in the day, a medical student was dispatched to purchase the zipper in a downtown department store, our own stock being depleted.

Can they do that? They can do anything.

I just heard a doctor say the lady in Room 32 is sick. How can that be? Of all the patients here, she's the sick one! It has an odd ring when a specialist in the ICU singles out a patient as sick. Something special is going on when medical terminology is turned in for the plain-spoken, something's beginning to unravel for sure, language first, as a formality.

Sick is for when your brother was not feeling well and was forced to stay home from school, so your mother said, don't worry, he's feeling a little sick: go on to school now, he'll be out playing in the backyard by the time you return.

"The lady in 32, she's really sick."

Which goes to show that context is everything, language is relative, and the relationship between signs and signifiers is unstable as a sixty-four year old smoker experiencing episodes of impressive angina pectoris, with T-wave fluctuation.

"Yeah, I eyeballed her when I came in, she *is* sick."

Surely they can come up with something better than that—what about a literature search, what's MEDLINE for?

"We can't do anything more for her…"

Now that she's sick.

A kid from Ontario with a breathing obstruction. Blond, a boy studying at McGill. I know those libraries myself, the stacks, and the humid cement stairwells. The Blackader-Lauterman: the art history library where I spent hours watching football games from the second-floor windows. Leaves scattered, red, yellow, and orange across the pitch. The players emit white clouds from their nostrils like bovine animals. And the furious play, a soundless spectacle, so familiar, from the windows of the library: the crowds leaping on the sidelines, players rushing deep into the end zones. A football, spinning, spear-hung in flight, describing a perfect arc from throwing arm to receiving arm.

They want to tube him. Laboratory tests show elevated liver enzymes, and so the usual questions are launched: have you ever used any IV drugs? He shakes his head, no.

Unprotected sex? Nods, yes.

Blood is drawn. We send away for the hepatitis ABCs and an HIV antibody screen. I hold his blood, three warm glass tubes in my wrapped fingers. Body temperature. Metabolism, a furnace. Condensation forms on the inside of the glass, something is alive inside there. Just below the black rubber stopper, there is a small window of opportunity for this reaction to take hold.

Blood. One of the lower classes of body fluids today, an untouchable, a caste below urine. Spinal fluid remains aristocratic, silver clear, pure as spring water. But blood has taken a beating. Yesterday it wore a cape, blood was valiant, vital, a bright, red metaphor for courage. The quarterback of life. Today blood is just another body fluid, dark, mischievous, heinous, sneaky, and untrustworthy.

"No Bloods on K."

Doctor's orders, they wrote them in his chart. Volume three. Usually they will request just about any test if a patient is heading downhill, so if a physician writes the prescription, "No Bloods on so and so," well, frankly, it's the kiss of death. From my perspective, that's how so many die here—from an order of No Bloods. The next day, when I come in, who had no bloods taken the night before, they are usually gone, off my census list.

They moved K from Room 50 into Room 46, a private room just across the hall from the nursing station. Another omen: being moved into a private room. As damaging to your health as an order of No Bloods. Done so family can grieve in peace and privacy the allotted few hours before our transport team is called.

K's two daughters and wife are singing their hymns again. It sounds beautiful. Full of beauty. The most moving experience that ever has happened to me here. Eerie. Perhaps this is the closest I will come to a nativity scene. I know he's dying, but the love, the respect, the serenity and calm of the figures surrounding him—their grief inseparable from their adoration of him in death, as in birth. I half expect the garish fluorescent lighting to dim and demonstrate a hardwired sensitivity in accord with the setting.

Mrs. K is about to become a widow, which might be easier to take, less abstract, than being the wife of a man in a coma. The daughters are singing more loudly now, near the end, no longer shy of us, between talking, between knowing what to say to each other and between silences, they sing over their father. They are burying him with songs, draping words and melodies over him, elemental as fire.

The son arrives. Daughters keep singing. Mother stands clutching her sleeve. A lone pillar holding no roof.

From the daily census, I read that K has been on the ward 108 days. Only J has logged more time in the ICU, clocking in at 140 days, and counting.

K's family are members of the ICU. They're part of the team. When K dies, what will they do with their evenings? Where will they go between supper and bedtime? All of us except K are on first-name basis. The daughters socialize with the staff, with the nurses and doctors, and they themselves follow every minor intrigue that happens on the ward.

An hour later, he's dead.

"Hi, Auntie? I'm phoning to tell you that father just died, we feel such grief, such joy ... you taught us so much about this ... we feel very alive ... we'll call when the arrangements are made ... Mom is here too ..."

The daughter with green eyes passes by my desk and apologizes for occupying the staff telephone line. I don't know what to say, I say it's all right. Then she walks back to his room, into the room of song.

The other sister comes to the desk. Dials a number. It doesn't work. I tell her to dial '9' first. "Oh yes," she shakes her head, "I'm forgetting everything."

She gets through. Her eyes survey the unit as she speaks, never resting long on any one thing. Our eyes collide and she smiles. So much love to share, she's whole, real, aware, giving of herself—giving now, a small sign, with her father in the next room.

"His spirit is filling the room. When I go out and then come back in, I feel it, it's huge and fills the room. It's strange and so powerful. We've been singing and crying and his spirit is filling the room."

MER

Hello.

Bonsoir.

How is it tonight? Busy?

Same as usual, not bad right now.

Sylvie working?

She's got time off.

That's right. I knew that.

What's this?

Possible hip fracture.

He fell?

Down the stairs. It's the weather, the ice. A 72-year-old male…

Allergies?

Penicillin.

Medications?

A nice collection. They're in the bag…

Sir, do you take anything for blood pressure?

Yes.

What did your doctor prescribe?

Medication, dear.

Which?

I take the pink ones.

These here?

I guess so.

Do you have any other medical problems?

I wear glasses.

That's good, you have a sense of humour.

Where are my glasses?

Under your stretcher, don't worry.

Are you sure? Where…

Sir, the ambulance driver put them in a bag underneath your stretcher. Anything else… only high BP?

That's what the doctor says.

How long?

Since I retired…

Are you in a lot of pain?

My leg…

We believe it's your hip, sir.

Then my hip….

Sir….

What?

We're going to take good care of you, don't you worry.

I have worries you've never heard of, dear.

That's good, you're a fighter. I like that. Put him in square four. Page Ortho.

Health care reform. Hospital closings. Rationing, restructuring, reengineering ... and here I am without a strategic plan to call my own, a human resource without a cause. A poster-child of the *virage ambulatoire*. One part overhead and one part deficit, I'm a Siamese twin, another worker bee made redundant by the cross-pollination of user-friendly spreadsheet software and the managerial class. It feels like, like a dream ... good as life was in the ICU, ensconced in my critical care niche, the hi-tech penthouse adjacent to the OR suites, someone took over my position upstairs while I was swept off the floor, down the stairwell, and slotted into the MER. The Main Emergency Room. The donkey's ass. That's trickle-down economics for you.

These are the trenches, the front-line of universal coverage. A live-action department, a 24-hour symptom-by-symptom telecast of human misfortune, misery, and mischief. I'm stationed in the Acute Care Area (ACA), a loud and bright intersection with stop and go traffic. A reception area for verbal abuse, a virtual thesaurus of chronic complaints, ranging from a two day old headache and garden variety nausea and vomiting, to a burning feeling when swallowing.

Alternate weekends, alternate Tuesdays and Thursdays, three-thirty to eleven-thirty shifts. At twenty-eight hours per pay, I'm a point two, part of the evening crew. My job is to keep a head count. Crowd control. Co-ordination, communication, and information dissemination. Some paperwork, my job is make up charts, stamp the stationery, and to help out where I can when I can.

All eyes all ears, I'm like Radar in MASH, I hear the ambulances incoming before the camera cuts to stock shots of the wounded.

We have people parked everywhere. Stretchers snake their way up the hall from the ambulance dock, around the nursing station counter and tail off down the corridor towards the swing doors that announce the Psychiatric Care Area. Gridlock. With no beds available in-house, no one's moving. The access ramps are congested. I just received a report of a four bed pile-up in the Observation Room. If you're heading into town with some dizziness, please remember there's a three-hour wait at the triage window.

And now for the news.

Patients are admitted, then stick with us in this purgatory over twelve hours, sometimes over the weekend, until we receive word of a free bed upstairs. Sick, tired, frail, or crazed, all together now. For these people it's something like having their day in court, outside, in the courthouse parking lot.

I was in the waiting room, pushing coins into the towering neon drink machine, when Mrs. B, the secretary from my elementary school, tapped me on the shoulder.

"Andrew, is that you?"

Twenty-five years since I was last dispatched to the principal's office. Mrs. B operated out of the front office. She doubled as the school nurse.

"I remember you, and your brothers *and* your sister…"

After so many years, Mrs. B was surprised to find me again, here of all places. Wasn't that lucky? Now, was I a doctor? Hopefully. Wasn't someone, my father, brothers, a doctor? She had read something in the papers. A nurse? Was I a nurse? A nurse would be nice, a nurse would suffice. No. Oh well, some kind of therapist, then? An RT, PT, or OT? What was my place and standing?

Could I sneak her backstage to see a cardiologist?

The hallway leading to the ambulance dock functions as a suburb of the ACA, an access ramp reserved for low priority cases. The people of hallway don't require continual attention, basically, they're in storage for a number of reasons. Down at the very end of the line you have the intoxicated teens and transients. They are joined halfway by the NYD group. Not yet diagnosed, these people have refugee status, but not, say, the rights of a rectal bleed. Finally geriatric admissions linger close by the nursing station. We keep a third eye on this group, old habits are hard to change and they've got plenty of them.

Taken together, as a unified group, these folks are the welcoming committee: when an ambulance arrives, the new cases are rolled through, their bed-on-wheels dividing a sea of spectators.

You too, they observe with mutual defeat. *They got you, too.*

The Emergency is a more powerful search engine than Yahoo, than Alta Vista or Lycos. Sooner or later everyone comes through the hospital for a visit. Accidents and illness cast a wide, wide net. Genetic inheritance hyperlinks with social behaviours and environmental conditions. Lung cancer's a click away from smoking. Smoking links with socio-economic class. And social standing hyperlinks with stress via control mechanism gateways, and stress with the immune system … alone or with family, as a guest or to accompany a friend, everyone comes through it's only a matter of time.

You can find anyone in here.

In the last month alone, we had the Polish deli-woman from up on the Plateau. I buy pierogis from her. She came in with her mother: angina. And we had the cook from my favourite curry house, delivered by ambulance: electric shock. The other weekend, in the Minor Care Area (MCA), I came across an old neighbour from down on avenue de l'Esplanade. Nothing serious: sprained ankle, left foot.

Build it, they will come: by ambulance, taxi, on crutches, in wheelchairs, propelled by their own steam or an unfastened seatbelt. Conscious or unconscious, blushed, jaundiced, or blue, here they come: film directors, pop stars, politicians. Those who live in castles carved into the side of the mountain, and those who in winter gather cardboard and nest on hot air vents downtown.

The poet Gérald Godin was here. Imagine: brain metastases. That was before my time, before I read *Soirs sans atout*. And Madame Sauvé, the former Governor General, she came in with something years ago. It's no state secret. One of these days Trudeau and Mulroney will show. Prostate, liver? Say what you will. And what about that actress who's doing the Pharmaprix commercials these days? She's not made of rubber.

This being Montreal, I'm waiting for Leonard Cohen to be brought up to us from a boat down on the river. For the intern from Saudi Arabia to touch his perfect body with her mind.

Here comes someone.

"Can I help you?"

"Yes. I'm looking for my wife."

A large man. He presses up against the counter, then pulls back and tugs his belt towards his chin. That's a sign. Like in baseball, when the batter steps out of the box, he's taking aim at me, the next pitch.

"Name please."

"F-I-L . . ."

Letter by letter, he's making it simple. Building a whole from parts.

"… E-M-O…"

It doesn't sound like one of ours. Maybe she was admitted, maybe she's in a clinic. Maybe she was sent home.

"I'll check in the computer…"

That's the best I can do, run her through the mainframe, though I see he's disappointed her name didn't set off any bells, that I work here, yet I'm not omniscient.

"How long does that take …Where do you think she is?"

He's drilling me now, applying a little pressure to keep me true. Nobody likes this routine, a computer mediated search, the client-server environment is not what it used to be.

"Don't worry. We'll find ..." Just give me a second here. "It won't take…"

The problem is, our computer records are never up-to-date. Day by day, yes, but hour by hour, no. The worst the system can do is list a dead person as a living person. Of eight bit characters, dead or alive, it knows no better than syntax strings, rosaries of zeroes and ones. A brief, digital afterlife is something we can all come to depend on, even sceptics.

"What time is it anyway?"

To hurry things along, he takes his car keys and ring and remote starter from his pocket and pumps a small green button with his thumb.

"When did she come in?"

"This afternoon…"

"Can you tell me why?"

Knowing *why* can tell me where, what clinic, which service, a number of things. But it's a high stakes manoeuvre like asking for a third card in blackjack.

"Head tumour."

Easy does it. Fine. That was close. It didn't throw him. He said head tumour like you might say third person, in a controlled voice, no quiver.

"I can't find her…"

I'm burning up. The atmosphere is not good. The Inquire By Name function draws me a blank screen.

"She came this afternoon with dizzy spells…"

Dizzy spells, seizures, they've been through it all.

"Was *that* her maiden name?"

I need more information, vital statistics, database fields and fodder.

"What do you … mean?"

I got him, cut to the chase: "What is her married name?"

He's annoyed.

"You use the *married* name here? You're the only … my mother died in this hospital and they used her maiden name. Aren't you guys supposed to use the maiden name?"

I lay down my mouse. I surrender. He's calling me "you guys".

"You're right … look, I agree, *they* should …" But don't confuse me with the creators, I don't write programs or design policy, nothing like that. You see where I sit, don't you? This is my office. I'm practically out on the streets. I come from the same place as you…we're of the same mind, given half a chance both of us would organise things better, we'd do it all over again so that you could find a woman with a head tumour by inquiring under her maiden name.

"If you need the married name, that's my name, it's Dimopo —"

Stop right there. Forget all about married names and maiden names: his is a Greek name, a twenty-six piece variation on three vowels, four consonants…

"How do you spell that, sir?"

"D-I-M-O…"

"All right. I found her…she's up on the eighth…take the elevator back down…"

That does it. He snaps his wrist—holding the remote, thumb poised over the green button. He's gonna self-detonate, would if he could. Nobody likes it when I tell them that to climb to the top floors, first they have to take the elevator back down to the ground and then, from there, cross over to a neighbouring pavilion and take a different elevator. Another setback, it's cause for a psychological grievance. Insult after injury. Final proof that, after diagnosis of a head tumour, nobody's opening any doors for them. Life couldn't be any harder, yet it isn't getting any easier. For some, being returned to street level is the last straw, a sinking spiral, the dizzy unravelling of cause and effect and emotion that lays the self bare as a hollow cardboard spool.

Sit up Mr. E. You haven't eaten. Have you had anything to eat?

Sit up, sir.

No.

Here you are. You need to eat, sir, or you won't get better. I'll push the tray closer to your side.

Not there!

Just a bit to the side, I'll move it over…

No. Shit. No goddamn…

Mr. E!

What the crap…

Can I help you Mr. E?

Yes. Yes all right.

He don't want it. He pushed it away.

Where's his family? You don't want to eat?

No, I don't want to eat.

They never come.

Can't you tell?

Are you sure?

Damn it.

We're trying to help you, Mr. E.

Yes. I know that. I know that.

Yes? You said, Yes!

Should I put your salad in a big plate instead of a small one?

All right…

Like this? Is that good?

No, not in there. Stop it…

He's never happy.

Don't let him get to you. Mr. E, what do you want?

He won't talk now, he swallowed his tongue.

Should I take his tray away?

Sure, go ahead. He'll just play with it. He won't eat it.

In late, I punch the combination into the lock on the men's changing-room door and enter between a row of brown aluminium lockers. George is trying on a red satin shirt. At least I think that's satin, deep, red satin, something from the wardrobe of Midnight Cowboy.

"Hey brother, what are you? A thirty-three waist?"

A second man, in a blue body-suit, throws me a pair of jeans. He's from Housekeeping.

"Thirty bucks. Levi's. Try them on my friend."

I've seen him around before, weekends, on night duty polishing the floors and emptying wastepaper baskets. When I started work here, it took me a month, a month of nights before I noticed him, his coming and going. He struck a different figure then, diminished, harnessed to his machine he passed through the hallways at the end of a thirty-foot electrical cord lead, in a parallel universe. But I see now that he's resilient to my imagination and blessed with entrepreneurial spirit.

"It's perfect. Thirty bucks is all I want."

My size, but not my fit. They do something strange to my bum, lift and separate.

"I'm not sure…"

There's no mirror in here, but I know how that feeling looks from behind.

"Free trade. No tax," Puts in George, the night orderly, trying to complete the sale for his friend.

The locker room is home to a ring of black market peddlers, roving wholesale suppliers, entrepreneurs. A hospital subculture that involves the housekeeping staff, co-ordinators, transport personnel, orderlies, sometimes nurses: just about anyone with a collective agreement.

"Thanks. But it's not me."

"Come back next week. I'll have some more stuff," the man in blue says.

"Can you order me a chest X-ray on Square 6 for unexplained weight-loss."

What's up Doc? I don't like the sound of that. As symptoms go, unexplained weight-loss is ominous. Square 6 is an open case. A team of doctors went over him dusting for lumps and swollen glands, and turned up nothing. All they have to go on is a gentleman who presented himself to the Emergency this evening, straight from the office, in suit and tie and polished shoes. He was meaning to come in last week, and the week before that, but he couldn't find the time. Work, family, commuting. A man who says he feels healthy except he's been losing "tons" of weight. I wonder if he had to punch a new hole in his belt strap.

Having no leads to follow-up, Dr. T must be fishing: for a mass, a growth, enlarged organs or constricted vessels, anything out of ordinary that shows up white on the X-ray.

"Do you want an abdominal series with that?"

These things usually come in pairs, as a combo like fish and chips.

"Sure. We better get one."

Unexplained weight-loss. He's over in Square 6 reading *Time*. Dark socks and his dress pants drain from under a blue hospital gown. He's intact, focused. He exudes confidence, an unexplained confidence, I would say, he secretes the stuff. My bet is, back in one of those glass towers downtown, he works a phone, splits his hours into minutes and cash-flow into capital without breaking a sweat.

93

Next up, John Doe. A male prostitute delivered to us by police escort, post-assault. The boy was discovered in a hotel room, face down, out on the town. A break and entry, police report he was broken into.

The triage nurse books him into Square 1, behind a pink partition curtain. He's a mess, they say, a pretty boy in a bad way. Cigarette burns to his face, cheeks, left eye lid. Broken finger bones. Hands are inflated purple oven mittens. Through a gap in the curtain I can make out a section of his right arm, an intravenous line descends from a pole and loops below bed level. He's plugged in.

A 28-year-old female comes in after baking a poison cake and eating it too. A brown poison cake. Looks like mocha. Bittersweet. No birthday candles. Two generous portions remain.

"Can they analyse this in Biochemistry?"

Dr. Q is asking. He's first year, middle class, a medical student. A hospital-system virgin. He hasn't crossed the bridge between textbooks and the guerrilla tactics of inner-city practice. This is his debut. A first date with the next thirty years of his life.

"They won't take it."

"Not a chance," George butts in from the sidelines, enthusiastic as ever.

The laboratories accept a wide range of products manufactured in-body: blood, spinal, and peritoneal fluid, and an assortment of low-end discharges and secretions, stool, urine, pus. But none of the labs, not Biochemistry, Hematology, not Microbiology or Parasitology, not Serology, Virology or Pathology, take poison cakes.

"Then how can I find out … she put in it?"

Dr. Q is persistent. But he's barking up the wrong tree, the torte is history.

George steps in to clarify: "If you send it up to the labs, *they* might eat it."

He means the lab technicians. They're undergoing contract talks. They'll stoop to anything.

Taking matters into his own hands, surely, as a preventive measure, George steps forward and retrieves the cake from the young doctor and slides it off the plate and into the garbage bin, job done.

"Poison cake," George turns my way, semi-thoughtful. "Where do you think she came up with that? Off the Internet?"

I shrug. Sounds good. Could be.

George sits down in front of the second computer, our spare.

"Does this thing have access?"

He pecks away at the keys and chases the mouse across the counter.

"How do you do it?"

George leans under the table, caught-awkward, head low, peeking through his knees, and switches the power off, then on again.

"What about Yahoo? Is Yahoo good?"

The Pentium revs up.

"So what do I search under? Poison, or cake?"

The global village idiot comes of age.

Status report. Square 6 rests: unexplained, a pheno-menon, an X-File. Still, he looks pretty good, loose, relaxed. And why not? They have nothing on him. He's not spooked. Not everyone is put off by this place. Maybe he's passed time in a Calcutta slum. He's seen worse, much worse. And really, compared to everybody else in the ACA tonight, he's a prize. Respiratory therapists just arrived to vacuum our fellow in Square 2. An echocardiogram was ordered on Square 4. That means heart trouble. And over in Square 1, our John Doe is receiving wound care. Two nurses are changing his dressings. Another soul, not far off, Square 3 or Square 5, is coughing à la mustard gas.

"I don't know what's going on with him."

Dr. T, talking things through with one of the nurses, Jane.

"Which one?"

"The guy over there, reading his magazine. He's lost more weight than Oprah."

"What's his history? Any pencil stools?"

Don't start with the pencil stools, please. They scare me.

"He's disappearing. He needs those X-rays."

George's partner wheels Square 6 to Radiology. He's in and out in fifteen minutes. That's rapid service. Developing, and a reading, take another quarter hour.

Marie delivers a fetus. A spontaneous abortion. She places the jar on the counter beside my elbow, a plastic specimen container with a pink twist-off lid, wrapped in paper towel.

"Pathology."

I nod, no problem, stamp a requisition and label the top.

"I've never seen one like this," Marie confides in me, "you should take a look. It's textbook perfect…"

I have nothing else to do, so why not. The fetus is undamaged, tucked-in neat, complete. Superficially, it is: textbook perfect. An architect's drawing, a blueprint. This is what the pro-life movement is about, this here in a jar. Dead cute. Suspended in saline, it resembles an astronaut free-floating in space, self-reliant, an umbilical cord for an oxygen line.

My wife is pregnant with one of these. We had the ultrasound last week. We're keeping the sex a secret. Our second child, we're set with sleepers, cloth diapers, rubber ducks, and a car-seat. I wonder now if we're jumping ahead in the game.

Marie leaves. She's working on the other side today. I lift the jar, careful now, and place it in the outgoing mail basket. Transport will pick it up shortly, and carry it upstairs to the laboratories. It's the weekend so they'll probably stash it in a fridge until Monday. Then, first thing Monday morning: technician, pathologist, coffee on their breath, scalpel, notepad, microscope. They'll treat the fetus to hard science, as they dissect their weekend.

At journey's end, it will not be recognizable.

The nurses have difficulty getting blood from John Doe, no veins, apparently. An intravenous drug user, say the Progress Notes. He was hitchhiking to Calgary, from Halifax. A cross-Canada work fair. Mid-journey, come to a fork in the road, he must have taken the path less travelled. The orderly found two ticket stubs in his pockets. Hockey tickets. A nice meal after the game? His story is being told, all night people are putting the pieces together.

"He's just a kid."

"His hair is dyed. That's not his natural colour."

"What a waste…"

Yet no one can fathom his world. The full physical exam turned up human bites on his torso. Bruised love handles. Burns up his arms, blisters cover his face, he's a medical history horror story, trade fiction. Holding court while two nurses change his dressings —this ruined majesty wrapped in a mound of blankets —he's a genuine mystery, enigmatic as the *English Patient*.

John Doe, who are you?

"He can't be 20 years old…"

No one is comfortable with the idea of him: a male prostitute. And all the cruelty that's gone on: cigarette burns, the broken bones, the force and drive of effort behind these outcomes. Who did this? Why? Where is mercy? He's let in a chill from outside, transported a little darkness into this bright clinical setting.

Disappearing, shrinking, something is eating Square 6 from the inside. A clump of cells, dividing rapidly out of control? In his lungs, a wad in his liver? It's a game of shells. Wouldn't it be simple if you could hold the man up to the sun or shine a flashlight through his tent of skin and scan his private wilderness of bones, tissue, organs. Of course, that's pretty much what's happening here tonight. An X-ray, a CT, an ultrasound. He's being developed, wavelength by wavelength, short and long, piece by piece, frame by frame like a roll of film.

His lungs, his liver. Heart, spleen, kidneys: who trusts these to keep them happy?

These circumstances reminds me of an adventure in de Gaulle airport. I was returning home from Paris at Christmas. High terrorist season. Line-ups and delays. Menacing overhead announcements. Paranoia reigned as passengers passed their hand luggage through the security machine, an X-ray box.

One passenger, call him Z, carried a large model aeroplane. An Air France 747. A gift, a souvenir. It didn't fit through the machine. Delay of delays. The airport security personnel tried every which way to pass the aeroplane through the X-ray, by stuffing it in backwards and sideways, one wing at the time, but it wouldn't pass. They struggled, persistent as Laurel and Hardy. Dogs were called in. And more X-Y chromosomes. Tough guys wearing thick blue, wool sweaters with epaulettes, and carrying petite automatic weapons. Again and again they tried to stuff the model aircraft inside the security box, to no avail. What began as a farce, deteriorated, humbling all those in the departure lounge, who watched grimly.

Pointing down the hall to an imaginary boutique, where, he had just, minutes ago, bought the toy, Z exploded into a rage, shouting, pacing, furious. Unshaven, dark skinned, and heir to the Customs suspicion of his geo-political profile, he was crying foul over discriminatory treatment. I had seen this before, in airports around the world, correlation confused with causation—cardinal sin of international and scientific communities—leading to the hypothesis of a genetic link to terrorism.

A man beside me, a fellow passenger who obviously didn't speak English, tapped my shoulder and made a motion with one leg and his hands and arms, illustrating that the model could be broken on one knee, its pieces scattered.

What's the fuss. It's dead simple.

I smiled and nodded my head, you're right.

Then, encouraged, holding my attention, the man pointed to Z and, in a second, violent motion, shoved his forearms down, jerked one knee, and broke his analogy in his hands.

You see what I mean, he nudged my shoulder, washing his hands in the air.

Z could be broken that way, over one knee, into pieces of small enough to be pushed through the X-ray machine.

And that would be the end of him, the very end of this nonsense.

Sordid, tragic, trivial. This is it—no allegory, no symbolism, no metaphor. I sit at my keyboard, slouched, I feel like Tom Waits, ordering bloods and X-rays, humming lines from "Invitation To The Blues." Unexplained weight-loss. Human bites. The kid's in there, through the curtains: a mound of white blanket, a section of his arm. He's quiet at the moment. No sound, not a word, or a whimper. The nurses tell me he's sleeping. Eyes swollen shut.

Poison Cake had her stomach emptied. Down here we get our share of post-suicidal gestures. That's what they're called around here, *gestures.* And suicide failures, we get them in too. That's as low as you can get, a suicide failure. A double loser. In six months of winter, six shades of Thanotos. The season of sun deprivation and discontent. February 15th is a charted peak on the graph, among teenagers. The day after Valentine's Day.

The first time I was dispatched to the Xerox machine to make a copy of a suicide letter, I remember the note was three pages long. Untyped.

I lay the sheets, solemnly, one by one face down over the glass. Holding the covering panel open, I watched the sliding shutter swing forward and back. A flash, and the paper borders, translucent, lit-up. A penumbra.

One copy for the psychiatry resident, one copy for the archives.

The last page was signed, "your sleeping princess." A glamorous description of a bulimic seventeen-year-old stationed in our hallway with a tube down her nose, vomiting liquid charcoal into a plastic kidney basin.

The handwriting was in a style I had seen before. Billowed consonants, and everywhere you looked bows and balloons instead of dots and crosses. I read the whole thing through and that's against the laws here. It was pretty plain stuff. I wouldn't call it confidential, average is more to the point. Muddled thinking, longings, regrets, a catalogue of misunderstandings. All those things that loom large in the mind of the beholder, larger than life.

I hoped for something more from a suicide letter, though I'm not sure why. Inspired brilliance, an epiphany. Perhaps, finally, some insight into truth—the human condition—an illumination from one so apparently close to death. But there was nothing there really.

Some spelling mistakes, misplaced apostrophes, incomplete sentences. Broken clauses.

The films on Square 6 come back. They are sent to us through the pneumatic tube system. I open the delivery capsule and pass the films on to Dr. T who clips them up on the viewing board, one, two, three, so that now again light shines through our unexplained man.

He is rendered in a blue-grey cloud emulsion, a triptych of indestructible plastic sheathes. Liver, lungs, kidneys. The usual suspects.

What's that? Maybe something *there*. Or *there*, staring out at us from inside the rib cage.

I can't see, I can't see: from the desk I can't see anything.

Dr. T unclips a film. He holds it overhead under the ceiling lights and stares through to the moon.

He touches his glasses, nudges them gently, using his thumb to push them back up along the ridge of his nose. Then he squints, scrunches his nostrils, and rotates the plastic sheathe 180 degrees.

Jane wanders over to have a look.

She cleans her glasses, while Dr. T sets the scene, with a word here, a word there.

He points to a far off star and she steps back into the clouds.

"My god," is all she will say.

Daddy look at me, look at me, who am I?

Who are you?

What is your name, sir? Talk to your daughter…

Daddy I'm speaking to you. Do you know who I am? Look I brought pictures of the kids. Look Daddy, look what I brought you. Daddy look at me and tell me what my name is.

Look at the pictures, sir.

They have to suction your throat, one more time Daddy. You'll breathe better.

Open wide sir. Open your mouth. I can't help you if you don't open your mouth. Open up wide as you can like at the dentist.

Daddy don't bite it. Just open up, one more time and it's over.

Open wide sir. Open up for the tube.

Wider Daddy, let him do his work. That's better.

Good and wide for the tube, sir, it's almost done.

Does it feel better Daddy?

It will be easier to breathe for you. We have to do that or else he's going to choke.

Good boy Daddy. I'm sorry. He doesn't like that.

Nobody likes the suction. Anyway we wouldn't do it if he didn't need it. He's going to feel a big difference.

I hope so. Do you feel better? That's the last time for today. Say Thank You to the man.

It's a loud kitchen, an open bar, a public square. An oral culture. In the old world tradition of storytelling, legends are passed along through the clan from storyteller to storyteller, from generalists to specialists, from A to Z up the hierarchy and back down. Every patient is worth a thousand words, and every service tells a different story, a variation on the theme, as information is relayed from paramedic to triage nurse, from nurse to medical student, and from the student to the staff physician via the senior resident on duty. All along, individual assessments are made and simultaneous exchanges occur, discrete elements are highlighted, added, revised, or deleted, and from a skeleton of medical sound-bites—CHF, COPD, Jaundiced, Hypoxic, Subphrenic Abscess—there emerges, at last, a taut narrative, a gem of economy and appropriate word choice.

I give you The Medical History.

In early, I pass through the waiting room and see two of our doctors in there, side by side, stethoscopes hung around their necks like gym towels, sunning themselves under twin television sets. It's winter so it must be hockey. Sunday, an afternoon game. A new time-slot for the Amerikanos. I catch the last five minutes of period one, then go in past triage and take my place in the ACA. The doctors stay behind and watch the first intermission, Don Cherry. Their loss, in a fee for service system, everyone's their own boss.

First impressions: it must be a dead day.

I'm right. The place is empty. The curtains are drawn to reveal six parked and denuded stretchers. Floors are clean, the air is fresh, no lingering odours or deaths. No ambulances in two hours, they say.

What's going on?

This can't last.

I anchor myself at the desk and coddle my coffee. To my left the orderlies are set, Tony and Jean are doing a crossword.

"Rembrandt's first name? Harmenszoon van blank. Four letters."

Jean asks the questions. Tony holds the pen. For some reason I think I should know this one. Then again, isn't Rembrandt, Rembrandt? Like Michelangelo is Michelangelo, like Pele is always Pele?

"A Gilbert and Sullivan opera. The blank. Eleven letters."

"*The Pirates of Penzance*?"

It's just a stab. I've been to Penzance, so there you go.

"Eleven letters," Jean mutters.

I've been cautioned. I better butt out, do my own thing. Crosswords coffee sit down chat, the evening develops. A work situation becomes a social opportunity. Who wants to flirt with me? A group of nurses are debating the pros and cons of owning or renting a dwelling. This dialectic leads straight into a series of familiar conundrums, a haunting discourse: To buy or lease a car? Private schools or public schools? Suburbs or city? A cottage in the country or yearly vacations down south?

Tony wants to order some food. Jean agrees. Pizza it is. The doctors come back in, we're losing 2-0. Thibault is useless. He doesn't cover enough net. He's too small to practice the butterfly style of goaltending.

"Have you ever seen him on the bench without his mask?"

Jean: talking to everyone, to no one in particular, to the group of five to eight, dispersed, grazing on magazines, somewhat organized around the nursing station counter.

"Next time, check out his hair...he looks like Tintin."

Jean never shuts off, down, but not off, like a clock-radio sitting in the corner on the kitchen counter, there's always something leaking from his mouth. He broadcasts a running commentary, one-liners tossed out like pucks onto the ice at practice, not all of them are picked up for play.

The evening resident for Medicine comes on at eight. He's a new face from an ancient land. A face from Egypt or thereabouts.

"It's a quiet night."

Everyone is reading, I welcome him aboard.

"I hope it stays that way…"

He indulges a timid smile. Sincere, nervous, awkward, he pulls his shirt out and tucks it back under his belt.

"I'm in Dermatology," he confesses. "I'm only on rotation for a month."

Well that's reassuring. I take his line about Dermatology to mean he's naïve in the affairs of the heart, the bowels, and the autonomic nervous system. Your average apprentice specialist, he's studying his bit of the body and operates on a finite plane. The liver is as foreign to him as the Red Army team of 1972. Just ask him to assess the mental status of an old woman with falls or to do a full physical on one of our urine-soaked transients, and he'd rather shovel snow all the way up University from Sherbrooke— with a tongue depressor.

Who among the living and the dead will serve the public good?

Another hour, no ambulances. Triage is quiet too, except for a Seizure and one lonely Chest Pain that made it up the hill. The boys are doing their crossword and the nurses have gone on to discuss daycare, as I knew they would.

I do what I always do here when I get bored: make a list. Tonight a list of T-shirt slogans.

Operate or Perish.

Cain is Able.

Your Condo or My Condo?

Homo Sweet Homo.

I Cleaned My Room.

Abort? Delete? Retry?

Cannibalism Sucks.

The Collective Unconscious is a Marxist Ideal.

Corporate Punishment.

I Love Child Labour.

Think Global. Drink Local.

Hands Off! I'm in the Control Group.

Who Among the Living and the Dead Will Serve the Public Good?

Our seizure patient had a CAT scan. A computerised axial tomography. A procedure, a technique: images of a particular depth in sharp focus, and deliberate blurring of structures at other depths for the examination of soft tissues of the body.

The films are clipped-up on the X-ray viewing board. Striking shots. Light shines through them, slices of brain, cross-sections from the gentleman eating a sandwich in square 5.

Clipped-up, no one is paying them any attention. The films have been read, interpreted, deciphered by the neurologist and radiologist, and now they hang, visual records, for the illiterate like me to gaze upon.

What do they show?

Layers, shades of grey, bones and skull appear white, air appears black.

An epileptic, stroke, possible tumour, lesion, mass, subdural bleed? Fluid accumulation, a cyst or swelling?

Was Square 5 frightened when an X-ray beam swept through his brain, along deserted neuro-pathways?

I see a crab beetle, a sword fish, the pleasing symmetry of mirrored hemispheres, a montage of ink blots. The Stone's album cover from the early eighties. *Emotional Rescue.*

There goes the phone. No. The fax. The ring is luke-warm, a warble, low-key, intelligent. Unlike the telephone which exacts obedience to a live speaker, you may defer a fax without it blowing up in your face.

From underneath the counter, the machine drones and out slips the transmission on limp paper that curls in upon itself. The facsimile paper, thin, smooth, pearl finished, is the quality of those role-out, mimeographed stencils that circulated in elementary school before the Xerox age. I remember the purple ink never dried on those things. Our math quizzes were set in wet. They gave off a pinching odour. After every math test my palms were smudged with a multi-layered print of multiplication tables, equations, equal signs, odd numbers.

Out slips the transmission, it goes something like this.

Mr. X, who was supposed to be shipped from New Brunswick to your Emergency Unit, via the Trans-Canada highway, died en route of a cardiac arrest, miles outside Campbellton. Our ambulance turned back, mission aborted. However, the wife and family of Mr. X, having left Campbellton by car one hour before the ambulance was set to depart, will be arriving at your hospital shortly. Please intercept them.

Intercept them? Look who went to Euphemism Academy.

Now things are heating up. I feel the urge to pee. I'm hungry. I need some positive distraction. What should I do? My feet are sweating. I put the paper down, pick it up, and read it over and once again I feel burdened by knowledge after The Fall.

I hand the dispatch to one of our ER residents. Julie from out west.

"That sucks."

She's going off duty. It's not her problem. She holds out the paper.

"Tell one of the other residents. Or tell a nurse."

Or go tell it on the mountain.

The neurology resident walks in. Square 5, the post-seizure case is his. Red hair, short sleeves, Richard from Hamilton.

Richard was down here a few weeks ago when disaster struck. A patient under his care turned sour. All of a sudden, there was an emergency in the Emergency.

"She's coning for Christ's sake!"

He ducked into the Resuscitation Room, and charged back out, raging: paged his staff, turned white. *Coning. Coning.* His mind was racing, you could see what he was thinking: *She's f… coning.* And it struck me immediately, that coning was probably one of those terms that means as it sounds, and it sounded to me like brain being squeezed down through a funnel.

Head trauma. Traumatic brain injuries. Read on: pressure builds up inside the skull, brain matter, swollen, swelling, bursts from its covering—its restraining tissue—and seeks release, free space. Enter the spinal cord: the last exit. Think of a hole at the base of the skull, instead of a funnel, and that's pretty much how coning was put to me.

She's coning for Christ's sake.

We have a wanderer, a lost sheep. He's here with his mother. She's having pain, chest pain, she says. But it's more complicated than that. For starters, she's on a rainbow spectrum of medications. Her differential is cloudy, cardiac versus golden age confusion. After listening to her side of the story, the department spin doctors have pinned her, an unreliable historian. She has cognitive deficits no program, no matter how aggressive, of debt reduction can address.

She's been handed over to Cardiology, who will assess her status.

EKGs are ordered. EKGs are done. Polygraphs.

The question is: is her chest pain sincere, impressive, angina pectoris, or some such brethren cardiac pain.? Or can the origin of her pain be found elsewhere: indigestion, musculo-skeletal? Did she, did she not, transport a cord of wet wood in her arms yesterday?

"What takes so long? We've been here for ages. When did we come in…?"

"It's normal."

Perfectly normal. I try to reassure him. He presses his hands on the counter and cracks his knuckles. He's not angry, just plain bored. Fidgety. Hours pass, as do his moods, through anxiety, anger, impatience, righteousness, frustration, a sliding scale that bottoms out on the side of utter and complete boredom: the system, you can't fight it, this is a no-time zone.

Hands in pocket, he wanders about, in a fugue state, oblivious, sweet oblivion, he no longer recollects why he came to this place, why he set foot here.

What's the attraction? He can't see it. Neither

can I.

Aimless, he comes to a stop in front of the X-ray viewing board and lifts his gaze.

What's this? Mother, is that you?

The viewing board attracts its share of visitors. A portrait gallery where you see pictures on exhibition: brain scans, belonging to our seizure man, and up beside them, chest X-rays—three of his mother— and several belonging to a newcomer, somebody known as a possible pneumothorax.

He feels he shouldn't stare, turns to walk away, takes two steps, then stops. He moves up close, nonchalant, shakes his car keys, makes some noise, he's not sneaking anything, everything's above board. It's not pornography, but something close to it. Indecent. A perversion of the natural. Shadows, white gauze-like outlines, ribs, lungs.

No harm done. No way he could tell lungs from the cerebellum, male from female, Picasso from Mondrian.

A team of doctors push in, surround him, blind to his presence they congregate, discussing histories and symptoms and test results. One of them keeps pointing to the films on the board, referring their attention away from his own interpretation and back to the pictures, themselves.

Three views of the chest. The staff doctor reads them like a television weather reporter deciphers a satellite slide, facing camera, light-pen indicating a pocket of free air caught between the chest wall and lungs. A pneumothorax. A high pressure system. Even

I know the remedy for that. Apply iodine to the area. Insert a chest tube intercostally, threaded just so far to rest in the empty cavity like a metal spout in a maple tree, and the air drains by itself. An X-ray post-insertion, another X-ray in twenty-four hours. And then you can pull it out and patch the hole.

Our man edges to the side and slips away, un-noticed, none the wiser.

1976. Time to pass. Grade school. I reset the question, pose the problem, anew.

X leaves the village of C travelling at a speed of G. P leaves C one hour before X and travels at the speed of Y. When did X leave C? How long before P arrives at the knowledge that X died of a cardiac arrest? How does P slow down?

Another hour, no one shows up. I thought the Campbellton bunch would be here by nine. Maybe I miscalculated. I'm going to fail. In any case, I've prepared my little speech for the family: Will you please follow me and wait in the family room and the doctor will come and speak to you when she has a moment.

I will stick to that line, deliver my syllables whatever the wife and family of Mr. X throw at me.

Another thirty minutes. Just one more hour and I get to go home.

The overhead bell rings. Someone's in the dock. An ambulance. Is it them? The doors swing open at the end of the hall. They roll up to the counter. Two attendants, one stretcher. I take my seat. The triage nurse receives them.

"This is a thirty-four year old male. He threatened his father with a knife. Untrustworthy. Watch it, he spits."

It's someone else. A violent spitter.

Jean disappears into the clean utility room and re-emerges twirling a blue surgical mask on a raised finger.

"What's his name?"

The man is fastened to the stretcher, three nylon belts tie his legs, waist, and torso. Only his head is loose, his neck rotates through 180 degrees of freedom.

"Alex! What's your name?" The tall attendant, shouting. "He doesn't know his name …Are you kidding! His name is Alex."

The triage nurse nods and Jean steps forward, main stage, and slips the mask over Alex, our spitter.

"He doesn't know if the rain hurts the rhubarb…"

The medics exchange glances, they like telling this story, they thrive on the attention of a captive audience.

"Alex who?"

The triage nurse cuts in, not interested in a turn of phrase.

"Alex D something. Here's his wallet. "

"Any money? Do we know this guy? "

The tall attendant checks his palm and recites Alex's address. He's got everything written down on his rubber glove. Alex's home address, his blood pressure, all his co-ordinates.

"Everyone knows him. He lives in your district."

Alex twists, his eyes shift. He's staring at me, straight into my eyes. He's taking down my number, whatever number that is.

"Come often?"

The interview takes shape. Medical history, past hospital visits.

"Weekends, holidays, Christmas. He's one of your frequent flyers. He does a lot of travelling in his head…you know, to buildup his air-miles…"

These guys have their act down, dead. They've been on this beat fifteen years. In the past, they raced stationwagons around town and flipped a light on the roof when traffic was heavy. Now that they drive armoured yellow tanks, they feel invincible, so they've become comedians.

"Call for his old chart."

That's an order for me, to ring up medical records and ask for the unabridged, complete works of Alex D Something.

"Did he cut his father?"

"No. His father went after him, then the wife called us. The police refused to respond. They know Alex…"

"Anything else?"

"Compulsive, strange behaviours and gestures."

"Does he talk? Is he oriented?"

"He says someone is trying to light his hair on fire. That's why he was spitting."

"Is that true, Alex?" The triage nurse glances in Alex's direction and continues on her way: "Any meds?"

"He doesn't take them. Although, according to our friend, he makes his own pills in his private lab."

"Where's that?"

"In the basement of his parents' house. But he doesn't take those ones either, he's very paranoid…"

"You just bake them, right Alex?"

The triage nurse finishes her notes.

"You can put him in square 3 for now. When Medicine clears him, we'll ship him over to the PCA, our psych-emergency."

The attendants deliver the goods into Square 3, then head outside. Ten minutes of happiness. And now it's back to the mean streets.

The night coordinator comes on and I rush to tell him about Mr. X from Campbellton.

"Figures," he says.

It figures, that sucks, what d'ya expect? It's become one of those worlds. A world of unsupportable attitude and debts to pop culture.

"They might not come," I tell him. "I bet they won't. If they're not here by now, they're probably not coming…"

He nods, he agrees. Sounds good, sound logic. The whole thing was probably just another fuck up anyway, right?

My shift is over, but the story of Mr. X has me thinking about my great aunt who died of pancreatic cancer four years ago. Eva lived in London, Ontario. That's an eight-hour car ride from Montreal, and an eighty-six year life-ride from Breslau, Germany, where Eva was born. I knew about Eva's diagnosis three months prior to her death. We were always close, but not close enough to touch and I couldn't afford to make multiple visits to London. Money, time, one of those equations. Even if Eva was dying, I had to *time* my visit, that is, I had to calculate, estimate, and choose the appropriate moment.

That same year, I was working on a series of prose pieces which I called *Translations*. They were modelled after Kafka's parables, which I admired, and, in fact, they were intended as translations of Kafka, but of pieces he had never written. You could call it "Ghost Writing." Anyhow, back then I posed the Eva problem this way.

If ever you have received word that a loved one, who lives at a distance from your home, is dying, then you may have set aside a moment to recite the following: Should I drop my things and leave on the instant? Or wait for news, and attend the funeral?

An interesting problem, posed as two questions. A tidy bit of writing, so I thought. Promising. I made slight alterations, revised, while I waited for news.

The psych-emergency is a sub-unit of the department, a six bed lost and found located down a back alley between the ACA and MCA. They have their own doctors and nurses, their own scientific journals and preferred drugs, celebrated diseases and sets of restraining belts. It's a whole different ball game. And not many people know how to play it. You would have to throw an orthopaedic surgeon a pretty big bone to get them to do a consult in there.

Our staff have a tendency to remark on the PCA —*our psych-emergency*—as if it were a Banana Republic among G7 nations, a developing country with a floundering tourist industry, undergoing intense counselling by the IMF. Psych nurses are frowned upon as being glorified babysitters, while, for the most part, psychiatrists must survive under the indelible labelling of *ineffectuals*, which rhymes somewhat with intellectuals.

As always, the division is between haves and have-nots, between a wealth and a poverty of cures: an illness that responds to treatment versus an unresponsive whole, an infection versus a depression, high-tech interventions versus talking cures. The difference is between having something to drain or surgically remove—a benign or malignant tumour detected in the inguinal area—and having to search, under rough conditions, for the black box containing the garbled flight-recordings between the pilot and the tower, lost at the bottom of the sea.

Medical history taking is the act of the getting the story right. Family and individual histories are recorded, revised, and edited by members of the multidisciplinary team, in the same way the synoptic gospels were transformed by the apostles. Apocryphal versions of an elderly male's chest pain are put aside as old charts are referenced and caregivers cross-examined. Retro-sternal pain turns out to be musculo-skeletal. A CABG in 1994 becomes a CABG in 1990. Unreliable historians are discredited, marginalized by diagnostic tests, X-rays, and clinical investigations and reports.

History taking is by and large a peer review process, a group effort, as one history is the culmination of several, or many, intertwining stories or accounts, originating from a variety of sources, not all of them reliable narrators: among caregivers, family members, neighbours, and referring physicians, some are given to exaggeration, some are of limited expression, while others yet are prone to metaphors and conceits, the magic realism of South American writers in the description of their symptoms and experience of pain.

My lungs are rainforests, bright green foliage dripping phlegm.

Doctor, a fern growing in my intestines keeps me dry, feeling dehydrated.

It feels like someone's pulling my hair when I open my mouth.

Report. Seven nurses, count them: standing, sitting, assembled in front of the board. Every eight hours, the nurses review cases, issue patient assignments. This time is called Change of Shift. This time is their time. You may not disturb them, like when animals are eating.

The magnetic board is the working memory of the unit. Magnetic strips are labelled with patient names. Differently coloured strips represent the medical subspecialties. Green for Surgery. Blue for Medicine. A round yellow magnet beside a strip means the patient is admitted. A hand drawn triton identifies a case for Psychiatry. An orange tag means Infectious Diseases.

Upon entering the unit, one glance at the board reveals everything: how the last shift went, how the next shift is going to shape up. Whether business is good or business is bad.

Before signing off, the day co-ordinator gives me the rundown. I'm debriefed by Rob. Rob's a lifer, he's been a co-ordinator about twenty-six years. It's all he knows. He can't be retrained now. Upon retirement from a place like this, after so many years of service, the staff get together and buy you a watch, a gold watch if you're lucky, which is not so subtle a hint: in the future, pal, make better use of your time.

To his credit, Rob's not doing bad. In part because he's managed to confuse sitting behind the front desk, day after week after year, with medical school. He wears a crisp, white lab coat as a mark of self-conscious aggrandisement, the same way I used to wear my new pair of Montreal Alouettes pyjamas around the house all day, on my birthday, and never wanted to take them off.

Report with Rob is serious business. He tells me the guy in Square 1 should have had an ultrasound but that *they* did a KUB instead. A KUB is a kidney-ureter-bladder X-ray. A big waste of time, a useless exam in Rob's view.

Secondly, I should *make sure* the lady in Square 4 is admitted to 5 Cardiac. Don't let *them* send her home. She's unstable.

The old woman in the hall needs her meds at eight o'clock, and the guy in the Isolation Room is booked for a total body scan. Nuclear Medicine will call.

By the way, the man in the Observation Room is dehydrated, somebody better order him an IV bolus.

Well that's it, he packs his thermos and coffee

mug, he's leaving now, but not without regrets—one last thing: *make sure* that lady goes up to 5 Cardiac. He gives his last orders on his way out and mumbles something about an arrhythmia. I figure he doesn't have the confidence to pronounce that one out loud, or he would use it, left and right, the world would know.

Sure thing Rob. You can trust me. The place is in good hands. I'm echelon five, practically a GP now.

Nuclear Medicine. That's a hard one to swallow, like Milton's *darkness visible*. An oxymoron, like chemotherapy. Whenever I hear Nuclear Medicine I wonder about Alternative Medicine. I have a friend who's a radiation oncologist. She admits radiotherapy has a frontier medicine image problem—that things like brachytherapy are experimental, if not alternative— and, given treatment outcomes, some forms of radiotherapy could be construed as palliative, as something complementary. Well, it depends on the disease group, some cancers are more sensitive than others. Of course. And she lets on, radiation is more harmful than anything a homeopath would ever prescribe, but not without citing things like controlled conditions and therapeutic regimens and ethical review panels.

She's right. I know she's right. Controlled conditions are one thing, over-the-counter herbal remedies are another—we agree—she's got me wrong if she thinks I lean the anti-establishment way—it all depends on what you're selling: hope, a miracle, comfort, a cure, your research, or your mythology.

"It's complicated…"

It is. We want to agree. Diplomacy is in the air. She wants me to see her as open-minded. And I want to be seen as rigorous, not ridiculous. So we say that when people are ill, when they feel sick and feel their sickness, they have a need, a right to feel treated. They have a right to hope, just as other people have a real need to prescribe treatments, to help, or to feel they are helping.

"When I was in New York, at Sloan-Kettering…"

Even so, the controlled conditions so often talked about make me think of the nuclear testing France carries out on islands in the South Pacific.

"Ah, but you're a poet," she says. And I know I'm disqualified, even as a third string bard.

"For us there is cause and effect, measurement and prediction, for you everything is simple, just drop a metaphor. For us there is a method, for you metaphor."

And for everybody else, I figure, there is both.

Square 4 doesn't have any bed sores. That's really nice to see.

What is she?

She's got some kind of paralysis.

Probably a stroke.

No. I think it was something since birth.

How do you know?

I heard the nurses talking.

She looks like a stroke to me.

It's amazing. Her skin is so nice, no ulcers, you know that's really nice to see coming from a Home. They must treat them well over there.

You have to be dedicated to do that kind of work.

You better believe it. I couldn't take it.

Which one does she come from?

A place on Sherbrooke, out east.

It's so rare, you know.

No kidding. Someone should write them a letter.

In late, I punch the combination, turn the handle and the door swings half-way open. I enter with my bicycle, bumping the front tire and catching the left pedal on the door frame. I'm stuck. So I push the door, but it's stuck too. Someone left a stretcher in here, against the wall. The door handle's caught on the metal railing. I start fighting with the door and the handle and finally I'm free, my bicycle too. I open my locker, throw in my helmet, and I'm just about to jump up on the bed to do up my laces when I notice there's a dead person under the blankets.

I pull down the sheet and expose the head, her face. Jesus. For a moment, I'm terrified, filled with dread. Then I recover: quit it, nobody killed her, she's just dead.

"There's a corpse in the men's changing room. A dead lady." That's the first thing I tell my partner Claire, at the desk.

"Mrs. G." Claire needs no introduction. "She died on us an hour ago. The family is coming in, they don't know yet … there was no place to put her… it's been crazy."

"We had to put her somewhere… we have no empty squares…that used to be the morgue…when the family arrives…"

Not another *when the family arrives* thing.

"…you'll have to get her out of there and find a place … where they can see the body…"

Sure thing. Someone in Resus will have to give up their bed though—I can arrange that, have the living and the dead switch places for a couple of hours.

They call out for blankets and sips of water and pain medications and doctors. Where is Scarlet? This unit resembles a civil war field hospital. A set from *Gone With The Wind*. They wet themselves waiting for assistance, holding out for a bedpan or wheelchair ride to the toilets. Where are the orderlies? It's not a place for the meek. The confused, the nauseous, and the short of breath, camp out atop flat black plastic mattresses. Elevated, on stretchers painted Caterpillar yellow, they're well situated to survey the staff in action, running circles, inserting lines, hanging IVs, administering pills, cleaning wounds, listening for bowel sounds, wheezing, or crackles. There's definitely no place out here to put Mrs. G, the dead lady.

Privacy is unique to V, who has been sequestered in the Isolation Room, the infectious disease suite, for carrying TB into our midst.

My company tonight is a middle-aged woman, dark hair, brown eyes, black jeans, leather boots. Clara. Clara's in with her mother: white hair, frail, confused, a case of General Deterioration. It's what cars suffer in countries where they put salt down on the roads in winter.

Clara's mother is parked in the hallway, propped up on scaffolding flush with the nursing station counter. Neighbours, separated by a half-wall, we could outstretch our arms and hold hands.

There's no chair for Clara to sit on. She stands to the side, out of the way but in the way, one hand on the stretcher railing—steady goes it, hers is a balancing act. Hand on the railing, fingers curled, she secures her mother's spot. Surely there's a queue? Observant, alert, Clara plays a subtle role: she distracts her mother when a man with a breathing obstruction is rushed through in a wheelchair.

We chat on and off about the state of the health care system and the government, taxes, the Expos. Current affairs. We compare ideologies. Share examples. She's read something about a new treatment for Parkinson's. And I have a story about my great aunt Eva who acted in a workshop version of Brecht's *Threepenny Opera*.

"That was in 1927 or 28," I say.

"It sounds so interesting…but I don't know much about the theatre…" Her voice trails off. Clara is busy doing the housework: while we talk she arranges the blanket for her mother, turns the pillow, adjusts the incline of the bed.

Clara's mother is quiet, a minor character in our conversations until, without preamble, the old woman stirs, and erupts from sleep, into Portuguese.

Mother and daughter are off discussing medications, the old country, and Clara's aunt's grandson, the doctor of the family. It seems every family has one. He's going to visit this evening and make sure everything's all right.

"My husband died here," the lady says, raising herself up, proud, pointing down to the ground beneath her stretcher. Then she slides flat, exhausted, though still talking with Clara, directing her voice upwards. It's work, keeping the conversation afloat, sending her voice up to her daughter, who is standing somewhere above her, to the side, out of view, hovering like a kite.

The two of them remind me of my mother and grandmother, my mother's mother, and how they used to carry on in Swedish and in English, unaware of any differences, fluent. And though I didn't speak Swedish, I understood something about the meaning it carried for both of them, and just by listening in, over coffee and pastries, I hoped to be playing a part in the survival of Swedish in our household. Many years later I miss its sound as much as I miss the house I grew up in, the very same house in which my grandmother is buried, inside my memory.

Clara looks my way. She's not forgotten me. She would include me if she could, but it's all Portuguese from here on in.

I feel comfortable outside their conversation,

nearby, but outside, minus a mother tongue I turn my attention to an old copy of *Vanity Fair* lingering behind the printer. The girl on the cover, wearing a blue-pastel sweater, is one of those supermodels. I recognize her super eyes and super bum and super legs.

I flee this world for another, for a kinder, gentler, more playful world of colour glossies, snappy articles, and teasing, low calorie recipes. A domain of browned buttocks, biceps, and breasts. Eye candy. Junk food. Something to munch on between answering the phone and ordering blood tests.

Clara interrupts. She needs a bed pan. I stand up and wander over to the clean utility room and return with a brown cardboard mould shaped like a cowboy hat. Prêt-à-porter.

"Hurry," Clara's mother pleads.

The old woman lifts her pelvis and Clara slips the cardboard tray underneath. The woman strains, sighs, and lets go.

"Don't worry. It's good Mama."

I do my best to disappear, shrink and fade, though I admire Clara, her vocal encouragements, her stance on nature's habits. It's not the time or place to be intimidated. Decorum won't do. If anyone should be embarrassed, it's not the elderly woman who must relieve herself in the corridor, surrounded by prying public and professional eyes.

It's good Mama. Go for it. Make yourself right at home.

I keep a low profile. *Vanity Fair*. Toilet reading. It

gives us each some space, this charade. I tune out and browse the bodies pressed between the pages, fabulous, voluptuous, bodies surviving decay, soft, unwrinkled surface area, from model to model no hint of deterioration.

Calvin Klein. Brut for Men. Eternity. Choose your scent. I open the sticky panels, they are like the tiny doors on Advent calendars.

A polite knock on the counter. I lift my eyes. Clara needs paper. Off I go and find them a roll. Then I'm back to my post at the front of the class, in a position of power, an invigilator perusing soft porn while two hundred undergraduates sweat it out over the Heisenberg Uncertainty Principle.

"Look after my mother," Clara half-pleads.

She's going home. I put away my magazine and sit up straight.

"She's exhausted." Clara frowns. Of course. Her mother's asleep. It's a small miracle. A tender mercy.

"It's a tiring place…you need your rest, too…take care of yourself so you can take care of your mother..."

I repeat these phrases again and again, night after night.

"Come back in the morning after a big breakfast…"

It doesn't sound like me, which, I know, doesn't prove anything.

They brought a man with heart failure. A native person. An aboriginal. A first nations man. An American Indian. An indigenous person. And no one knew what to call him.

Sixteen weeks pregnant, 16 years old. Assaulted. Blows to the head, kicked in the stomach and brought to us under police escort.

"O my god, O my god!"

She's buckled over in pain. Jane kneels beside the wheelchair and rubs her back, massages her neck.

"Page Obstetrics!"

Tony grabs hold of the handles and wheels the assaulted pregnant woman into Resus. That's where people are taken when it's serious business, out of sight, into the Resuscitation Room.

"May I…"

The police officer, two-hundred pounds plus, asks formal permission to use the telephone, as if it were the last chocolate in the box.

"Dial 9 to get out."

The officer puts a call through to the station. He settles down, bareback on a black swivel chair: facing backward, stomach leaned into the cushion, legs astride.

"…we got his name… one of her boyfriends who hangs out around Berri and Ste-Catherine…"

Tony emerges from Resus with some bloods.

"CBC, Sma7… and they want an Ultrasound …"

Diagnostic tests, clinical investigations. The medical team is building their case.

"Stupid fucking bastard she's in labour…"

Flustered, Tony drops the blood tubes in the basket and returns to Resus.

"Is that a murder, if…?"

I swing around, the police investigation is underway.

"Put me through …"

The officer is put on hold. He cradles the receiver on his shoulder and begins doodling on his report sheet.

"Coffee?"

I point to the kitchen.

"Fifty cents."

He transfers the receiver to his hand. He's got someone on the line again.

"…if the baby is born dead, is that manslaughter?"

I see his angle now. Murder, manslaughter, assault and battery?

"What's the number for Legal Counsel? Can you put me ..."

I stand up and get the man a coffee. He's got a job to do.

Coffee, cream, sugar. He nods, leans back on his horse, acknowledges my service. And when I go home in the evening, I think: that's what I did tonight, I bought a coffee for a man investigating a murder.

Settled in, first thing I make a list: order food trays, call in admissions, clean up any outstanding X-rays, fill prescriptions. I number each item and draw small square boxes, aligned perfectly, that I check off, one by one after each task is completed. I keep this place in order, organized, I run a tight ship on paper. My list is my illusion, a diagram of the anatomy of my shift. Symbols, numbers, and boxes aligned on the page. A translation once removed from reality. A coping strategy.

Life: growth, metabolism, reproduction, and adaptation. A mode of existence. I never thought of it that way. Clever, neat, conceptual.

Vegetative life: a set of programed, automatic acts. The body as it maintains only the essential services: fire protection, police, air traffic controllers.

C with breast cancer, with mets, spreading through bone and skin, arrives from the ODC. Oncology Day Clinic. With cancer nothing is safe, not your tibia, not your children, not your dreams.

Relapse is the word, it follows remission. Her cancer returned after she hoped it was gone forever. She's read the literature. She knows where she stands, on which slope, on which distribution graph.

Her daughter is silent and furious. She can't believe it.

Her son, twentysomething, joins them, persecuted by inadequacy—what can he do to help his mom? The boy is imploding.

At least I know where to find a straw when the daughter asks me for one, some action taken, finally.

Here you go, I say, take two, knowing already they've drawn a short one.

Surgery. Medicine. Psychiatry. Here stands a hospital, a house divided. Scalpel, stethoscope, fountain pen. Anaesthesia. Antibiotics. Anti-psychotics. Table, bed, couch. Surgery. Medicine. Psychiatry. The synoptic gospels, a trinity: the father, the good son, and the holy ghost. Clean the area and remove it. Rehydrate and observe overnight. Tell me about your childhood.

To live or die by the sword. To live and let die. To be or not to be.

Surgery. Medicine. Psychiatry. A tumour. An infection. Voices.

Jeff's in the house. The night orderly. He comes on at eleven, singing something, rap, sounds like Whitey on the Moon.

"Waz-up?"

He acts black, which he isn't, but so long as he doesn't start calling me *bro*, I won't blow his cover. Why spoil things, it makes him happy. He has black-envy, no heavy crime in style appropriation.

"Nothing much…"

He deposits his money belt on the counter and unclips his pager. He's got two. One for work, one for personal calls. If only the doctors were as obedient to their pagers.

"Cool man … catch you later…"

Look at him go: he rolls with attitude, his neck and shoulders have been fused together by hours spent working machines in the gym. Who says they have it tough in some other countries. This guy, and many like him, get thrown between a steel vice every morning and have to pump their way to freedom and a protein milkshake. He told me himself, he's bulking up. He's got a five-year plan. And already, he has those thick bloated arms that resist straightening, held from his trunk as if an electric field of some sort kept them that way, floating, cocked, and stiff as if about to draw.

Jeff's quiet, he works hard, never causes trouble. Everyone says he's good with patients.

Good with patients. You hear that all the time. A doctor who is said to be good with patients is somewhat like the family dog that is good with children. An orderly who is good with patients, like Jeff, is an orderly who is gentle with the scrubbing and rubbing and doesn't treat the meat like meat. Nurses rarely receive the same verbal treatment, since it is assumed, fairly or not, that all nurses are good with patients. However, nurses can be said to be good. As in, he's a good nurse. She's a good nurse. Now *there's* a good nurse. Meaning, technically sound on top of the soft human stuff.

Dr. W emerges from the Resuscitation Room and flips a chart into the outgoing mail basket.

"Home. Allergic reaction."

I reach for the chart and retrieve the carbon copies, sign and date the discharge slip, while Dr. W continues around the counter and passes behind my chair.

"Page Cardiology."

He speaks into the open air Dictaphone that I am, stream of consciousness ruffled by terse, bulleted commands.

"Make sure Square 8 gets a chest X-ray…"

Got it. I dial up locating and wave the requisition at one of the orderlies to get things going.

Dr. W takes his seat over to my left, beside a medical student who has been waiting patiently in the wings. Her name is Teresa. We met earlier on. Teresa's from Boston.

"So who do we have here? Let's go, we only have a few minutes before rounds—who do you have?"

"I've got two."

Teresa has two prisoners.

"Let's have it."

The straight dope. Just the facts. Dr. W wants to clear the deck.

Teresa begins: "An end-stage male of Latin origin, AIDS related, closest kin unknown … picked up on a park bench. And I have a woman with a brain tumour who is known to this hospital and followed by one of our cancer guys."

Cancer guys are Oncologists. Oncologists are male or female.

"Which one needs immediate care?"

"Neither, really. I don't think."

"You don't think what? Let's go. Rounds in ten minutes. Tell me, in your opinion, which is the shorter case… less complicated . . . "

"Probably the brain tumour lady. She's a reliable historian … followed by this hospital, she has an old chart and her story is well documented."

"I see. Good. And the other case? What's he running for?"

What are his symptoms, what are the slogans? Essentially, who will admit the patient? Surgery or Medicine? That is the question.

"…um…"

Flat-footed, Teresa mumbles something incoherent. She's lost. This is her third week. She's not entirely fluent in the language of this 'hood. Dr. W is, he's got street credibility. He continues on course, weaving his best solo good Doc, bad Doc routine: "…is he a strong candidate for Palliative Care?"

Will he win the election?

"*I* think so."

Teresa drops the I-bomb (*I* think so …) to indicate she has a mind of her own and that it might not be working properly.

Dr. W unfolds his hands on the table and says nothing. He waits. Teresa makes a note. Maybe Palliative Care was not such a good idea after all.

"What are they doing these days with respiratory

infections? Do they go to Medicine—to the Chest Hospital? Who takes them?"

She's backtracking. He's the expert. The ball's back in his court.

"It depends. Page Medicine."

Dr. W wants reinforcements. I page Medicine.

"...it really depends on the bed situation and the gatekeeper..."

The short answer. The Bed Situation and The Gatekeeper deserve whole chapters of explication. Now is not the time. Back to the decision tree of knowledge:

"Now, first: is he comfortable?"

"He's breathing rapidly. We put him on oxygen."

"Anybody home?"

Is he orientated or confused? What's his mental status?

"He's in and out. He's on fire."

He's slipping in and out of consciousness. He has a high fever. Teresa's picking it up quickly, they're jamming.

"How high?"

"Low forties."

And with freezing overnight in the low-lying areas.

"Immune system overtime."

Good grief. We're into extra innings. The sudden death format. These two are going to break my heart.

"He's really burning. Will he have a seizure?"

Now that's something I would like to know myself. My daughter spiked a high fever over the weekend. She was panting, delirious. We didn't know what to do.

"…probably not. You won't see that."

That's it for febrile seizures. Dr. W won't be up for the annual teaching award.

"Now what about the other woman, does she need attention? What's her story again?"

Teresa starts over: "A 59-year-old female with a brain tumour followed here and across the street, was found outside the gates of Club Price, post-seizure."

"Isn't it Price Club?"

Dr. W is sharp, so sharp.

"That's what the Urgence Santé notes say: Club Price. I don't now. I'm not from around here…"

Dr. W: "…those guys can't spell … no, I think it's Price Club. What do *you* think?"

They want a third opinion. My nonsense worth.

"What do *I* think?"

There goes: I drop the I-bomb and dive for cover.

The echo is inevitable: "What do *I* think?"

I wonder which came first: italics or phonetics? What do *I* think? I don't want to say what I think. Leave me out. Anyway, I say Club Prick.

"So what about this lady?"

Dr. W is back on track. Forget Price Club. It's a red herring. Rounds in five minutes.

Teresa: "On exam, nothing too exciting. Bruises. Some minor abrasions."

Did I hear minor savings?

"Is she oriented now?"

"She's fine. She has a swollen ankle. The left one.

It's pretty bad. She must have gone over on that side…she's a big woman…she needs an X-ray. Otherwise as I said, a brain tumour."

"Okay. That's fine. You can present her in rounds. We still have a minute or two. Let's go have a look at her, together."

He stands, she stands. And off they go.

Sunday. A quiet beginning. Report, change of shift—only five items on the menu. The board is clean. Three green strips for Surgery, one blue for Medicine, and another, orange, for Infectious Diseases.

Helene is braiding Jane's hair. The nurse in charge has new shoes. Someone else wants to get a pair. How much did they cost?

People are noticing things. Smelling the roses.

One of the orderlies is offering massages.

It's a touchyfeely time. A mood is set. It's sunny outside so no one is coming in, death and disease have the day off, they are out enjoying the weather, taking air with the rest. Nothing keeps people out of the Emergency like a sunny afternoon in early spring. Nothing brings them in like October rain clouds, an ice storm, or the St. Patrick's Day parade. The after-hours parade route ends here, in a racket and a stink, a series of stretchers at the far end of the hall assembled in line like floats.

A group of nurses arrive late, in civilian clothes they're transformed: pleasant, casual, athletic. Radiant. Full bodied, physical. Looking like they haven't been sick a day in their lives. Like every organ and extremity is getting all the oxygen they need. Sunday nurses. They look like Sunday nurses, out for a drive.

They come bearing gifts. Designer coffees, ultra-white Styrofoam, high vaulted plastic lids. And bagels and cream cheese.

They've just dragged themselves in from a brunch: a bourgeois affair, the eleven o'clock secular Sunday service.

Now look what the kitchen staff just dragged in: a metal caboose, the food truck. I call on the overhead for the orderlies to distribute the meals. Hospital food: toasted crushed wood, neon vegetables, meat that sweats. Elmer's white glue soup that sticks to your ribs and teeth. The orderlies work quickly, open the truck, three doors, eight shelves, it holds about twenty trays. Hurried yet with considerable care, they slide out the trays, place them on trolleys, every motion measured, calibrated, so as not to spill, so as not to touch.

Here comes someone. A young male, baggy pants, fat striped orange T-shirt, black toque. Could be a Point Zero mannequin.

"My grandmother dirtied her bed."

I need an orderly. The sheets need changing. The lady needs a washing. The family want to see it happen now.

"Why didn't anyone notice? If we didn't come in tonight, when would you guys have noticed?"

Watch it, any second now he's going to blow his cover as a cool, no-sweat hipster, I've seen it all—from Mountain street to Crescent—from the cockpit of my JEEP 4X4.

"I'll get somebody right away."

The customer is always right and around here the customer is always dissatisfied. In theory you can talk about priorities of care and limited resources, emergencies versus maintenance strategies, a breathing obstruction versus soiled sheets, but in practice there's no excuse for this kind of thing.

"Let's hurry it up, please."

The family member glares back down the hall where the rest of the clan is waiting. There's a handful of them, all ages, children and adults. This one is their ambassador.

"It's disgraceful..."

They came in tonight to visit their mother or grandma or aunt and discovered her lying, trapped, in a wet bed. Right then they must have frozen. No one's moving, even now no one can talk.

"I'll get someone..."

I call on the overhead for Jean or Tony.

"Orderly to Acute Care, please. Orderly to Acute Care."

Seconds later, my call is answered overhead by another speaker.

"I'm stuck in ..."

It's Jean. Tony's on break. Jean's stuck somewhere, probably in the MCA, outfitting someone with crutches. I didn't catch everything, he got cut off by locating.

Locating rule the airwaves. After the bell, now, the locating girl speaks:

"Code blue 7 Medical. Code blue 7 Medical."

There's been a cardiac arrest on 7 Medical. Code blue is the resuscitation code. It means: patient turning blue. Talk about priorities. The crew with adrenaline and two charged hand irons lead the rescue. An in-hospital commando unit, the cardiac team parachute behind enemy lines, pounce, and revive—further questioning of the dead.

"Code blue, code blue 7 Medical…"

The locating girl's voice is clear, calm, somehow sensual, a controlling and soothing anaesthesia. Code blue, code blue: voice of a siren. Who is she? The omniscient narrator. She knows everything. Sees everything. Locating locates. Locating knows. Omniscient, non-judgmental, any married man could tell her all his secrets and she'd understand. Nothing excites her, not even a cardiac arrest. Locked away in an office behind an unmarked door, the locating girls, as they are collectively referred to, operate a hospital-wide virtual conscience.

The family member is waiting at the desk, watching me watching him. He won't budge. I call again on the overhead to prove I mean business.

"Orderly to Acute Care, please. Orderly, please…"

My mate answers, this time I hear him.

"I'm down in Room 4. Five minutes…"

Just as I thought. Room 4 is in Minor Care, the plaster suite.

To be thorough, formal, and polite, I relay the message to my friend, although he must have heard it himself.

"It will be another five minutes."

He looks at me like I'm insane, some stupid asshole. I'm the impotent bureaucrat and he's the guy kicking against the bricks. We're both nothing but method actors. I wish Jean would hurry up. Every whole second grandmother lies in pee, soaking, is a slow, ticking, insult.

Rattled, feeling vulnerable now, I almost throw in the line about the Health Minister. Everyone is saying it these days: if you have a complaint, and really want to make a difference, write a letter to our Health Minister.

The Health Minister. Now there's an abstract target.

"Look it, you better get somebody …"

Now I'm beginning to lose it. I don't like feeling this way. How long will these folks wait, I wonder, before someone, anyone, his sister or nephew or niece face up, take things into their own hands, and do the deed. We're not talking about defusing a smart bomb here.

"All clear, 7 Medical. All clear 7 Medical."

A false alarm. Good enough. The cardiac team may rest easy.

"What was that?"

My man is pricked by the last overhead call.

"Nothing. They just called off the code."

Rest easy, pal. No one's trying to pull something over on you.

The overhead call system is instrumental to getting anything done around here, useful, yet disruptive. Pages, codes, general announcements—the bell-tone, the voice. Has anybody studied the effects of the locating system on in-patient treatment outcomes? If you're nauseous, confused, then I bet it's all just noise, bewildering, destabilising as those police tactics whereby agents surround fugitives and drive them out of hiding by turning loose a Black Sabbath box-set at full volume, set on repeated play.

Jean comes up the hall.

"What do you need?"

The family member stares. This is him? This is the specialist we've been waiting for? This cleans my grandmother up?

"...a bed changed ... in the hall ..."

"Let me wash my hands…"

Jean drifts away, into the clean utility room. The family member clears off from the counter, slowly, tight-muscled and stiff, unconvinced. His body language sits with me another twenty minutes.

Today we're squeezed in, under siege, overrun and outnumbered. The working conditions are not working conditions. And ambulances keep coming. Low on linen and vacant stretchers, there's nowhere to put Them. The experimental group is spilling over into the control group—they are becoming us, we are becoming them. A mutiny is brewing as standards of care slip. Who's accountable? The staff feel betrayed by administrators and under appreciated by the public. The public feel neglected by staff, forsaken by government. And the government sits with frozen books, accountable to none and all. That's the virtue of a vicious circle, it keeps going round, a snake swallowing its own tail.

Hostility, condescension, guilt, frustration, finger-pointing—it flows both ways, back, forth, up, down, like a fever trapped inside a thermometer.

"All I do is flop, it's lousy for my circulation. I'm miserable. You should all go home ... release me."

The voice comes from the other side of the counter, down a bit to my left. Mrs. H. A sensible woman, from what I can tell.

"This is an endurance contest ..."

Her voice is persistent yet resigned to not being heard, or taken seriously, a monologue rising and curling through itself like second-hand smoke from an ashtray.

"If I was home ...this is what they did last time when I was here, I lay here, lay here, and lay..."

She's not imagining things. She's been lying in the hall all day, last night she spent in the Observation Room.

"...who is my doctor?"

Who is she kidding? That's a question I truly dread. It's almost as ridiculous as: where can I find a wheelchair? We don't have many of these things. They went out with the care in health care.

"Do you have a doctor or do you not have a doctor?"

Now the doctor comes. So we do.

"I want to go home. Please let me go home ... you're already full as you are, give someone my spot..."

She's altruistic, or masochistic.

"Believe me I'd let you go but you had a stroke and things are not right. The notion is you should go back on blood thinners tomorrow morning."

Things are not right...? The notion is...? Where

does he come from…the notion is he's a wet noodle, indecisive, non-committal as a divorcee.

"I'll take anything. Blood thinners, cod liver. I was in Britain when they bombed and it was better than this. I can tell you there are places better than this. This is a ghetto."

The gatekeeper cometh. Quiet on the set. All rise for the Grand Inquisitor. Gatekeepers are imbued with mythological status, guardians of the Cabala, they possess magical powers, control the silk route and regulate the ebb and flow of hospital admissions and discharges.

The gatekeeper is received with awe as it is rumoured that he *has beds*. Has beds, hasabeds, hasbeds. Whisperwhisperwhisper. Could it be? Where did he get them? Open beds. That rare commodity: a free hospital bed. A mattress, clean sheets and blanket, a pillow: in a room, with a nurse and doctor? And the support staff to cover all the bases: a matrix of helpers, water carriers, and maintenance people.

Open beds? Take us to your leader. We'll trade him muskets and communion wine.

A balding man in his fifties, the gatekeeper is human after all. This month it's the flamboyant Dr. S, a jolly, efficient, eccentric. Tonight he sports a pair of black, anti-embolic, spandex cycling shorts. He's on his way out. His mountain-bike is chained to a lamppost outside. He's nouveau-young. Strapped over his shoulder, he carries a leather side-bag. His trade-mark. What's he got in there? Unfilled admission orders, a sandwich, an oil can? I've never seen him open it up.

He arrives in bright spirits, loud and energetic, he rounds the counter and hollers a general hello.

"How many do you have for Medicine?"

He waves the nurse-in-charge over to the desk.

"My dear, how are you tonight? And who is the

doctor-in-charge? My niece is looking after the kids…"

Our staffman spots Dr. S and hurries over, after disentangling himself from a family member.

"We've got seven for you. I'm totally wiped…"

"Seven? Good lord! Seven for Medicine…"

Dr. S spins around, chattering.

"We better get a move-on. Why didn't I get a call earlier? This is crazy…who is first? Who is … lucky?"

Dr. S extends his hand to one of our geriatric admissions who has spent the holiday weekend in the hallway, ferried to and from Radiology, stationed with a view of the dirty utility room.

"Anglais ou Français? English or French?"

The language question. You can't escape it.

"What did you say?"

The man speaks up. He's English. Let us give thanks. For now, we are spared Dr. S's French.

"Hello. I'm Dr. S. The gatekeeper. I need to ask you some questions."

A mental status report is what he's after.

Dr. S: "Where are you?"

"Here."

"Where is here?"

"In the hospital."

"Which hospital?"

The man yawns.

Hint: The Royal Vicious Hospital. I try to feed him my answer. No good, the buzzer goes. Next question:

"Who is the Prime Minister of Canada?"

"Which one?"

"It's a simple question, no trick. Who is our Prime Minister?"

The old man smiles, mildly, ambiguously, like when new-borns release gas.

Dr. S turns up the volume: "Is it Pierre Elliot Trudeau?"

The man is transfixed, so is the staff. I hear grumbles. My friend Marie from the Gaspé winces.

"Is it Brian Mulroney?"

"No!"

"Sheila Copps?"

He purses his lips, and blows, sharply, a small dart.

"... who?"

"Could it be Jean Charest?"

Silence. Suspense. I'd say that's a trick question.

"Yes."

Resignation replaces smiles. Next round of questions.

"Take 2 away from 100."

"68."

"Take 2 away from 50."

"18."

"Take away 2 from 4"

"20."

That's the buzzer. Time up. The gatekeeper leaves his contestant to go and confer again with the Emergency staff doctor.

"This man is totally spaced out. He's totally off on his own…what is his history?"

"Basically, he came in confused, hypoglycaemic ..."

The staff pauses to review his notes. "He's been wandering around my whole shift…I haven't got to him, yet…"

"That's it? No fever?"

"…he was down on the totem pole, so I haven't seen him …"

"Doctor, take away 2 from 60."

"Very funny. It's been a night to remember…"

"Well, this man is not with us. We'll admit him to 6 Medical and shine a light into his attic, upstairs."

Princess Di is dead. The GI resident brings the news.

"She had an accident and the guy died too."

The guy and the driver and the princess. A royal mess. The staff is dumbstruck. I don't see why— tragedies are played out every shift right before their eyes, yet they can't get used to this: the death of a princess, a random hit minus a biological perpetrator. It feels make-believe, or stranger than fiction, a grotesque mix of fairy-tale and objective fact. Cinderella assassinated on the way to the ball. Who would dare?

I decide to take my break out in the waiting room. Everyone is glued to the sets, even those, I imagine, gripped by their own, immediate health concerns.

A reporter confirms everything while witnesses parlay their disbelief. Princess Di is dead in Paris. Life's every form is fragile, the world is not a safe place, not even Paris. Whereto now romance? Events like these inspire acts of introspection in the most unlikely of individuals. Take the orderly tonight, he says, "You'll be shown her face from century to century but you'll never see her alive again."

I shake my shoulders.

"It's the truth, man."

Everyone has their angle, a theory, something they call their own philosophy. My grandfather used to say: Life is a great teacher but it kills all its students. He told me he read that somewhere—the human condition, elusive as intellectual property rights.

The neurology resident waltzes in carrying a small, black leather handbag. He's here to tune the piano. Press keys, check the action, elicit notes, reflexes, involuntary bodily responses is the game. Equipped with art deco hammers, prods and pricking devices, neurologists perform the most elaborate rituals. The formalized physical exam resembles an exorcism. They play the nerves, feel for muscle tone, manipulate limbs, palpate, touch, hold, orchestrate the motor and sensory pathways.

They knock on tendon just so, with panache, using a metal stemmed hammer with a triangular, rubber head. The tomahawk.

One brisk tap, quick and direct.

Ding.

In a symphony they would play the triangle.

Otherwise, there is something of the archaeologist in this doctor type. The instruments of their trade descend from the same branch of the tool family, hammers, prods, picks. Moreover, they share a fascination with minutiae, an intellectual adventure revealed in the study of human antiquities. The digging, excavation, sifting through sand and tissue, through layers, the tireless search for fossils, origins, relics, markings, imprints, abnormal structures or growths.

Lesions, bleeds, ceramics, arrow heads, papyrus.

The lunch room, staff room, our bunker: a tired couch, a few chairs, dim lighting, microwave, a fridge jammed with Tupperware and Rubbermaid, a radio and a low coffee table strewn with *People* and the *Order of Nurses Quarterly* and an assortment of hospital leaflets, memos, and pamphlets, generated by the politburo. The staff cram in on their breaks to read complain browse eat bitch nap. It's this place or the ambulance dock, there's nowhere else to go. We talk about nothing, about the same things we talked about last shift, last week, last year, budget cuts, constitutional issues, Seinfeld, about a certain rude, married doctor and a certain kind, young nurse. We pass the time, tell stories about our children. Boyfriends, girlfriends, husbands, wives, mistresses, lovers. And yes, we go on about the pension fund and the baby boomers, and about the ageing population with such dire familiarity you would think we all kept one or two down in a room in the basement. As though, my goodness, our elders—who treated us all to ice-cream—represented the next great threat to our social security after the Asian economic flu.

A man is wheeled in from triage and raced into the Resuscitation Room. He's conscious but I guess that could change. Acute chest pain. Unstable. History of a triple bypass graft.

Call the bomb squad. STAT. Cardiology.

Slow down, don't tip him. He looks in bad shape. I hate chest pains, they make me anxious. Even the medical staff will handle a CP with excessive care, lift him slowly from the wheelchair onto the stretcher, bare his chest and apply electrodes here, here, here, and here, for an electrocardiogram. Next an X-ray, next a blood gas, next the cardiology resident, fourth year, loads of experience, long, shining, auburn hair.

She makes medicine look easy, like something she does everyday after brushing her teeth.

She plugs into her stethoscope and lowers her head down over the man's chest.

Tick. Tick. Tick.

Shush.

She's picking his lock, his safety deposit box. She takes the man's hand, it flops like a fish. She holds his wrist, thumb over the artery.

"Hi, Andrew," she says, spotting me in the crowd.

She smiles, blows her hair out of her eyes. She can't talk now.

Do you have any of the old mechanical beds?

Why?

We got a guy coming from OR, over 400 pounds.

Come on…

He'll break the electric beds and the new ones go for five grand a pop.

Are you serious, he's over 400? There goes my back. I'm on in the ICU this weekend.

We'll need the crane from the stadium.

What did he have?

They tied his tubes, a gastric something.

How old is he?

Under thirty.

He could make an animal go extinct all by himself, if he liked a certain meat.

You should call in sick.

I'm going to. There's a game on, too.

When a taxpayer passes away, John, Jane Doe, I dismantle their chart and send it down to Medical Records. I ask one of the orderlies to bag the corpse and I call for the transport team to come and collect the body and deliver it to the morgue. It takes about an hour, door to door. After that, it's anybody's guess. It depends on your beliefs.

Next I clear them off my computer screen.

"Are you sure you want to discharge this patient?"

Ever watchful, the system software prompts my next action. I draw a line with the light-pen, a slash through "yes".

"Thank You. Patient X has been discharged from your census list."

The last words are programmed.

Take five plus ten. I step outside for my break. A bag of salt and vinegar chips. I need to get away. Outside the garage, the ground is littered with cigarettes. A tobacco stew, tar meets tar on a hot humid night in July. Ambulances come and go. Thirty-one degrees and the city has cement breath, heat rises, time-released, from the core.

I walk out to the top of University and look down over the city. Buildings jut up from the central basin, aglow, towers clustered like disposable flashcubes. It's been an evening of strange behaviours, beatings, and verbal abuse. A summer fugue. A festival of primal urges. *C'est fou. C'est le bordel.* A psych patient propositioned me with a butter knife. A drunk visited the waiting room with a steel bar. Then came the arrival of a woman by ambulance, postpartum, post-coherent, her new-born was found by the police tucked away in a dresser drawer.

I have these fifteen minutes to get away. I check my watch, view the city from above. I'm seeking some perspective in a very literal way. A new-born in a dresser drawer. That's no NICU. A dresser drawer, Jesus, son of Mary, stranger things have happened. Resurrections, resuscitations. In the distance on bridges draped over the river, a chain of red lights signals the outbound traffic. Electricity's brocade. I follow their progress, commuters retreating to the suburbs, the South Shore and beyond, into a wilderness of population statistics … of morbidity rates and demographic profiles … my attention lapses, I check my watch again and by some paralysis of will I cannot read the time.

The clock-face reports back esoteric detail.

I stare, my eyes migrate over the city, from light to light, shining, shining—never assembling sight.

I forget what I'm doing.

The clock-hands wing forwards, at blind intervals, and then, at the very moment time is told, they hold stiff like a butterfly pinned under the glass.

I've been gone over twenty minutes. I'm late going back in. Ready or not, here I come.

I take a walk down to the Observation Room to deliver a message to Mr. U. He's got the place to himself, no bunkmates.

I knock before entering, the door stands ajar.

No response. But I know he's in there. I can hear something. A mice-in-the-walls kind of noise, rustling paper. I've disturbed him, surprised him. This is how it is when I play hide-and-seek with my three year old, Sonya. She hides under the blanket and squeals when I enter her room. I have to pretend that I can't find her, stall, while she readies herself to be found.

I hold up a second, here in the doorway on the threshold of Mr. U's room.

"Hello," I call, from my side of the partition curtain, "guess what?"

Now, upon entering, that is, standing inside the room proper, I realise my ill-fortune. I have come upon a micro-climate like one of those sunspots you pass through swimming in a pond. The air is thick. The odour, pervasive, heinous.

"What's that?" He calls out, disoriented. Mr. U's engaged. I sent Tony in here to deliver the portable potty about an hour ago.

"You've been admitted to 6 Medicine. You're going up…"

173

I like bringing good news, and what better news than this: Mr. U is going up. It's like when Radar finds out Trapper's going home, back to the USA.

"Oh, that is good …wait a minute there …"

He's hurrying things up.

"Take your time, sir…"

Mr. U stands, I hear the lid collapse.

One minute, he's doing up his gown. Those things are impossible to tie—a short string, a knot behind the back, fine motor skills. They are not Parkinson's friendly.

"I just had some diarrhea…"

Diarrhea is something that happens upon you, an intrusion. In my house we used to say that too: *I just had some…* as if diarrhea came out of nowhere and used the premises as a mouthpiece, like an oracle.

"Can you get me another one of these?"

He waves a sanitary napkin through a gap in the curtains, a white flag gesture.

"I'll get you some toilet paper, sir … I just wanted to tell you you're going up …"

"Fine …but can you get me some more of these? They work … best …"

Adaptation is the story of evolution, I suppose.

"Someone help me. Please help my son."

I rose from my chair and registered the image. A mother and child. Terror, love. Panic. The boy was heaped in his mother's arms. Wet laundry. Legs hung, limp.

She came rushing into the ACA past the triage window and then stopped, holding the boy for everyone to see. No sight of blood, no trauma. The boy was struggling, semi-conscious, moaning, trying to escape some awful thing. Whatever it was, it was internal.

I have a girl that age. I was a boy that age.

People rushed forward from all sides, nurses, orderlies, myself. This is a hospital for adults. It was disorientating. Everyone rushed to help the woman and her boy, not actually to treat, but to help, act, to come to their rescue through any means, professional or unprofessional, clustered around the woman, around the boy, so much good will and raw feeling.

"He'll be all right. How long has he had this fever?"

This fever, of course. A fever. That's it, he has a fever. A nurse took the child from the mother and led the group into the Resuscitation Room. She held the boy upright, one hand supporting his head on her shoulder.

The mother held her hands to her mouth and followed, some paces behind, evidently relieved to have the boy taken away from her, off her hands, though not out of the woods yet.

"Dr. D. Resuscitation Room. STAT. Resuscitation

Room. STAT."

The mother began reciting a story as the boy was put on the stretcher. He had a fever, a high fever for days. She was going to bring him in yesterday. She thought it could wait, wait and see was the plan. She didn't know what to do.

"Tonight I panicked. My husband is away…"

She jumped in the car and started driving. She had him in her lap, driving, he was getting worse, she couldn't make it another minute.

They swabbed the boy's forehead. He was held down, in place, on the giant bed surface so he wouldn't roll off the edge onto the floor, a distance twice his height.

Dr. D arrives. Looks like a febrile seizure, he says, let's give him some acetaminophen.

"Page Paediatrics."

He's not sure about the dosage, the boy's weight. Children are not his bag.

Paediatrics give us a call back: "What the hell, who do you have over there? You better transfer him…"

I go back to the desk and call for an ambulance. I sit down, stand up. I can't keep still.

A few minutes later, I'm called back in.

"What's going on?"

"Hey, Andrew, come here…"

Dr. D is holding a syringe loaded with the liquid pink.

"We can't get it in..."

I see it's been a group failure. They've been

praying, hoping for it to go in. This is strange. They've been caught off balance by the boy and his mother. I've never seen this before.

"Don't you have kids…"

I do. I know the routine. This I have done. I must be the only parent on duty tonight. I look around the room. None of them have children, and they call themselves professionals.

I held the syringe and cupped the boy's jaw with my other hand. After two years in the Emergency, this was as close as I'd come to another human being. *Here you go, this will…* I pried his mouth open, and poked the syringe in past the gate of his teeth. He struggled, even in his fevered state he knew his boundaries, sensed violation.

I held the boy upright and squeezed. The boy swallowed and almost immediately his jaw slackened, he relaxed, and I gave him some more.

The mother thanked me. I wanted to thank the boy.

Following the patient and family interviews, the clinician sights land in the prospect of the physical exam. Solid ground, tissue, blood, bones, body-parts that do not speak. Organs and non-sentient systems. The initial diagnosis based on a traditional story-line fleshed out with stock symptoms, is deconstructed when the physical exam produces unsuspected details, and in these, unforeseen evidence of a second assassin.

Enlarged lymph nodes. Swollen glands under the armpit.

Treatment plans change. The picture turns cloudy. Consultations follow in rapid succession. GI, ID, Medicine. The conventional narrative is subverted by post-modern techniques, a multiplicity of voices, footnotes, texts, and subtexts. Of truth, there is none after all, only stories, different versions of the same event, a differential diagnosis.

So you see: after an inauspicious beginning, the plot thickens. Caregivers grow silent. Family members bite their tongues. A suspicious genetic inheritance ties in with egregious social behaviours and events develop through complications to a catastrophe in which there occurs a sudden reversal of fortune.

178

See *Tragedy: A Glossary of Literary Terms*, 5th Edition, M.H. Abrams.

When a brave soul, in a timid I don't want to bother you voice, requests permission to go home, straightaway, forfeiting medical care, he or she is ignored, low priorities yet troublesome, their appeal is received with suspicion, with a hostile blend of indifference, arrogance, and impatience, even wounded egos.

How dare they ask to leave us and forsake medical advice? Once you're in, you're in. And that goes for everybody.

The party line will not serve them. Only those well enough to be sent home, would dare utter such a request. Meanwhile, there are, please notice, some sick people who require our immediate care. Therefore: don't bother us now. Sit tight, count yourself lucky. Stop complaining. Take a number.

Remember the lady who had clubbing?

…from last night?

I did a CT this morning and she had mets.

Excellent job, man.

It's my first real diagnosis. And another guy I did last night had something in his left lobe.

It's in the air this weekend. I'm telling you man, it's nuts.

I know. It's true.

Cool, see ya. I'm going up to the ICU, they did a valvoplasty on one of our guys.

So much depends on four valves of the heart: the tricuspid, pulmonary, mitral, and aortic.

My shift is over. I'm done here. It's almost midnight. To leave, I have to pass through the hall on my way out where stretchers line up head to toe, alcohol abuse to confusion post-seizure to abdominal pain NYD. Passing through is like walking the plank, they'll try to stop me, stare, and by the time I make the doors I'll have been judged and sentenced, and self-sentenced.

Before I get going I take a moment to gather myself together. All set then, let us go, I zip up my jacket and prepare my face for the faces I am going to meet.

Someone needs to go to the toilet. A man requires help to get out of bed. Another is thirsty. An older woman is cold. She's lying under the air vent. The fan is driving her crazy. She needs another blanket.

Don't they know it's change of shift? I'm going home.

Where are the orderlies? The orderlies should take care of these people.

The orderlies are busy.

It's me or nothing. The bells toll for Thee. I go for a blanket but draw the line at a glass of water. You don't give money to every panhandler on every street corner do you? Of course not. It's no different here.

The man who is thirsty looks out of sorts, like he's been whisked from a chimney. He reminds me of a street person, whatever that is. More likely, he's pre-op. Booked for an emergency surgery, he's been lingering in the hall without a shave, without food or his glass of water. I bet he's NPO. He's not allowed anything by mouth.

When I pass his station, he reaches out from atop his stretcher, one arm crooked he waves me over with all the urgency and drama of a killdeer leading a predator away from its young ones.

I don't want to know what I don't know. I lower my head. It's my dignity or their dignity. I avert my eyes.

Afterword

The ICU is a perfect workspace for a writer—bright, quiet, controlled—and it was there, behind the co-ordinator's desk that I set down, on hospital stationery, rapid sketches and the first drafts of *Wardlife*. I remember being jealous of the nurses and doctors on duty, of all the time they spent writing—okay, charting—while I looked on, stranded between a telephone and the three-hole puncher. It wasn't long before I began doing my own writing at work—vignettes, dialogues, fragments, notes, poems. At the time, I considered all these as practice pieces, finger exercises, since my intent was only to hone my skills as a writer by working quickly, committing to paper what came across my plate, in whatever form suited the immediate moment. These were to be snapshots, still lifes, études. Hence the book's subtitle, *The Apprenticeship of a Young Writer as a Hospital Clerk*.

All of these stories, or sketches, as I like to call them, are based on real events, on things that I saw happen, on episodes that actually did take place. Yet they are stories, meaning my first loyalty has been to the narrative, not to record facts and figures. For the latter you would have to look in the hospital charts. However, I do believe these pieces accurately depict life on the wards, the language, the culture, as well as the current 'crisis' in the delivery of healthcare in our hospitals today.

To use an old standard, sometimes I have lied to tell a truth. Sometimes, as in the passages to do with my own life and family, I have used real names and kept to historical facts. All other names are made up, while the characters given play in these pages are composites and represent personality types, not individuals.

Andrew Steinmetz
Montreal
October 1999

www.vehiculepress.com